LESSON I
FOREWORD

In this book the writer thereof seeks to convey to women—particularly to young wives and women expecting to be married—certain important facts of knowledge, certain necessary information, which all such women should possess, but which few are given the opportunity to acquire.

It would seem to require no argument to convince a rational individual that before a woman is capable of intelligent motherhood she should be made acquainted with the physiological processes which are involved in the sexual functions leading to the state of motherhood; but we are confronted by the fact that few young women are given such instruction.

It is a strange thing that while even the ordinary school child is made acquainted with the physiological processes concerned with the processes of digestion, respiration, circulation, elimination, etc., and while such education is highly commended, yet at the same time not only are the young of both sexes reared as if there was no such thing as sexual functions in existence, but even full-grown adults are left to pick up their instruction on sexual subjects from chance sources—often polluted sources.

Even those about to enter into the important offices of matrimony and parenthood are permitted to assume those duties and responsibilities without intelligent and scientific information or knowledge being given them. What would we think of expecting a woman to cook, without previous experience and without even the most elementary instruction on the subject? What would we think of expecting any person to undertake any important task or duty without experience or instruction regarding the same? And yet we seem content to allow young women to enter into the important relationship of marriage, and to undertake the important office of motherhood, often in absolute ignorance of the physiological processes involved, and the physical laws governing the same.

All this absurd practice and custom results simply from the antiquated notion that it is "not nice" to speak or think of the subject of the sex functions. The subject has been considered "taboo" by our particular section of the human race since the Middle Ages, because the ascetic ideals of that dark period of human history brought forward a totally false and unnatural conception of sex as fundamentally impure. If the results were not so deplorable and often tragic, this condition of affairs would be a fit subject for laughter and scornful ridicule. But, alas! on the part of the thoughtful observer of this state of things there is rather great wonder and amazement accompanied by the feeling of deep sorrow.

It cannot be honestly denied that in our present age, and period of modern civilization, and particularly among the Anglo-Saxon branch of the race, the question of the sex functions is associated with impurity, at least so far as the popular mind is concerned. In previous civilizations the subject was accorded its proper place, and was discussed sanely and thoughtfully, without any sense of shame or impurity. The Middle Age ideals of celibacy and asceticism brought about the public conception of the human body as a thing impure—something to be modified, tortured, subdued and reviled; and a corresponding conception of sex as a vile, impure thing above which the pure in heart rose entirely and completely, and which those of a lesser spiritual ideal were permitted to indulge with a due sense of their degradation and weakness. It was considered a most worthy thing to lead an ascetic life with its accompaniment of disdain and punishment of the body. It was considered most pious and spiritual to forego the ordinary human relations of sex, marriage and parenthood. From these distorted conceptions naturally evolved the idea that sex, and all connected with it, was a subject unclean and impure in itself, and to be avoided in thought, conversation and writing. Not only the ordinary sex relations of human life were placed under this taboo, but also the phenomena of birth and parenthood. Not only did these incidents of life grow to be considered impure, but they became that which to many was still worse, that is to say, they became to be regarded as "not respectable."

Ignorance regarding the plain elementary facts of sexual physiology is undoubtedly the cause not only of much immorality among young people of both sexes, but also of many unhappy and inharmonious marriages. The intelligent portion of our race is now beginning to realize very keenly the fact that the first requisite of sane marital relations and intelligent parenthood is a practical and clear knowledge of the physiology of sex; education concerning the sexual organism, its laws, its functions, its normal and healthy conditions, its anatomy, its physiology and hygiene.

The average physician of experience in general or special practice can tell tales of almost incredible ignorance on the part of young women who have recently entered into the relationship of marriage. In some cases the ignorance is more than a mere absence of knowledge—it consists too often of false-knowledge, untruthful ideas concerning matters of the most serious import. It is sad enough to think how such persons may work results harmful to themselves, but it is even sadder still to realize that these same ignorant young women must eventually gain their real knowledge through sad experience—experience paid for not only by themselves but also by their children. It is a hard saying, but a true one, that the knowledge of many young wives and mothers is to be gained by experience paid for by their (as yet) unborn children.

The writer of the present work is one of the rapidly growing number of thinking persons who believe that the time has come to educate the race concerning the importance of sane instruction concerning the functions of sex. He, and those who think as he does, believe that the time has come to "Turn on the Light!" They believe that the importance of the subject will be realized by all intelligent persons, once that their attention is directed to the subject, and once they have considered it apart from the old prejudices and distorted customs. When public opinion on this subject is reformed, then will the taboo fall away from the body of truth; then will the subject take its place among the "respectable" topics which may be considered, discussed, and taught, without loss of caste or prestige.

In a few decades, perhaps even much sooner, it will be regarded as quite reprehensible to permit young persons to enter into the relationship of marriage without a sane, practical knowledge of their own reproductive organism and the functions thereof, and of their physiological duties to themselves, to their companions in marriage, and to their children born or to be born. We may even see the practical application of the somewhat startling prophecy of Newell Dwight Hillis, D. D., who said: "The State that makes a man study two years before a license as druggist is given; that makes a young lawyer or doctor study three years before being permitted to practice; ought to ask the young man or young woman to pass an equally rigid examination before license is given to found an American home, and set up an American family."

While the information above alluded to should be given alike to the young husband and the young wife, it cannot be doubted that the latter is the one of the pair who is most in need of this kind of instruction. While both the young man and the young woman require this instruction, the need is the greater in the case of the young woman, by the very nature of the case. The sex functions and processes play a much more important part in the life of the woman than in that of the man, the protests of some of the modern feminists to the contrary notwithstanding. The careful student of the sex life of men and women frankly confesses that in both the physical and the psychical realm the sex offices make a greater demand upon the time and attention of the woman than of the man.

The love-life of the woman is far fuller and more absorbing than is that of the man. Unhappiness concerning her love-life renders the remainder of the life of the average woman of comparatively little account; while, with a happy love-life she will put up cheerfully with the absence of many other things which are usually regarded as necessities for happiness. As a writer has said: "Essentially, a woman is made for love—not exclusively, but essentially; and a woman who has had no love in her life has been a failure."

The same rule operates on the physical plane. As the same writer has said: "Physically, the woman is also much more cognizant of her sex and much more hampered by the manifestation of her sex nature than man is." The manifestation of the incidents of menstruation is a constant reminder to the woman that she is a creature of sex. The phenomenon of pregnancy is, likewise, something from which the man is free. And, finally, the menopause, or "change of life," with its incidents greatly influencing the physical, mental, and emotional well-being of the woman, is Nature's final word to the woman that she is the active pole of sex-life. As the above-quoted writer has said: "Altogether it cannot be denied that woman is much more a slave of her sex-nature than man is of his. Nature has handicapped woman much more heavily than she has man."

And so, in this book, the young woman—the young wife—is directly addressed, her companion and mate being referred to only indirectly.

LESSON II
ANATOMY OF THE FEMALE SEX ORGANISM

Every woman should be given plain, practical, sane, sensible instruction concerning the sex organism of woman, its functions, its laws, its use, and its abuse. This important feature of the physical organism plays an all powerful part in the life of every woman, and particularly in the life of the married woman. It is nature's mechanism for the reproduction of the race. Every child that is born into the world is conceived, gestated, and finally delivered as a result of the functioning of this organism. Therefore, such instruction and knowledge is vitally necessary, not only for the intelligent performance of the duties of parenthood, but also for the best interests of race-preservation, race-culture, and the physical well-being and health of the individual woman.

And yet, custom and ancient prejudice have drawn the veil over this most important subject, so that it is difficult for the average woman to find practical, clean information concerning her own anatomy and physiological functions concerned with her sex-life. To many it has appeared that the particular organs and parts of the body concerned with the reproductive functions of the woman are base, unclean, and impure, and that any woman discussing them, or seeking information regarding them, must be immoral or at least not "respectable." Anatomical charts and physiological treatises on the subject are tabooed outside of the doctor's office. Women are considered immodest if they seek to acquaint themselves with the facts of life concerning one of their most important classes of physical functions. It is considered "not nice" for a young woman to know anything about her physical being in those phases which play the most important part in her life. Can there be anything more ridiculous and insane? This is a matter which excites the most intense surprise, disgust, and despair in the average person possessing a scientific tendency. But the dawn is breaking, and a better day is ahead of the race concerning these things.

The sex organs of the woman are divided into two classes, as follows: (1) The external organs; and (2) the internal organs. Let us consider each of these classes in turn.

THE EXTERNAL SEX ORGANS OF THE WOMAN.

The external sex organs of the woman are as follows: The Mons Veneris; the Labia Majora; the Labia Minora; the Clitoris; the Meatus Urinarius; and the Vaginal Orifice. The term "the Vulva" is applied to the external sex organs of the woman in general, but more particularly to the Labia Majora and the Labia Minora (the larger and smaller "lips," respectively). The term "Vulva" is the Latin term meaning "folding doors."

The Mons Veneris is the fatty eminence or elevation just above the other external organs, which forms a mount from which its name (literally, "The Mount of Venus") is derived. At puberty it becomes covered with hair.

The Labia Majora are the large "outer lips" or folds of skin which enclose the Vaginal Orifice, and which are situated just below the Mons Veneris.

The Labia Minora are the small "inner lips" of folds of membrane, which are concealed within the Labia Majora, or "outer lips," and are seen only when the latter are parted.

The Clitoris is a small organ, about an inch in length, situated at the upper part of the Labia Minora or "inner lips," and usually being partly or wholly covered by the upper borders thereof. At its extremity it has a small rounded enlargement which is extremely sensitive and excitable, and which is the principal seat of sensation in the woman's sexual organism.

The Meatus Urinarius is the orifice of the urethra of the woman, the purpose of which is to afford an exit for the urine. It is located about an inch below the Clitoris and is just above the Vaginal Orifice. It is a common error among uninformed women that the urine passes out through the Vagina; but this, of course, is incorrect, as the two canals and their respective orifices are entirely separate from each other, though situated closely together.

The Vaginal Orifice is the outer entrance to the Vagina, or Vaginal Canal or Channel. This orifice is located just below the Meatus Urinarius. In the virgin it is usually partly closed by what is known as **"The Hymen,"** (vulgarly known as the "maiden head"), although in many cases the latter is absent even in the case of young girl infants. It was formerly regarded as an infallible sign of virginity, and its absence was regarded as a proof that virginity was lacking. But this old superstition is passing away, for science has shown that the Hymen is often absent even in the case of young children and infants, and, on the other hand, is sometimes present after several years of married life, and even during pregnancy. Much unhappiness has been caused in some cases where the husband has doubted the virginity of his wife because of the absence of the Hymen, but consultation with a capable physician usually removes this misunderstanding.

The Hymen is a membranous fold, sometimes circular in shape, with an opening in the center, though in other cases it extends only across the lower part of the orifice. The opening in the center is for the purpose of allowing the menstrual blood and the other secretions of Uterus and Vagina to flow through. In a few cases this opening is absent, the Hymen being what is called "imperforate"; in which case the girl experiences difficulty when menstruation begins, and a physician is required to make a slit or opening in it. In some girls and women the Hymen is quite tough, while in others it is very thin and is easily broken. In the latter cases the young girl frequently breaks the membrane during vigorous exercise, such as jumping rope, etc. And, as has before been said, in some cases infant girls are born without even a trace of the Hymen. Under the circumstances, it is seen that the presence or absence of the Hymen is far from being an infallible proof of the presence or absence of virginity, and the belief in the same is now regarded as almost a superstition of the past.

THE INTERNAL SEX ORGANS OF THE WOMAN.

The internal sex organs of the woman are as follows: The Vagina; the Uterus and its appendages; the Fallopian Tubes; the Ovaries, and their ligaments, and the round ligaments.

The Vagina is the canal or channel leading from the Vaginal Orifice to the Uterus or womb. It is situated in front of the rectum, and behind the bladder. In length, it averages from three to five inches; and it curves upward and backward, reaching to the lower part of the neck of the womb, or Uterus, which part of the neck is enclosed by it. It is a strong fibro-muscular structure, lined with mucous membrane; and is not smooth inside, but is arranged in inner folds or rings which are capable of great extension.

On either side of the Vagina, near the outer orifice, are two small glands, about the size of a pea, which secrete a peculiar fluid, and which are known as the Glands of Bartholine. The office of the Vagina is that of a complementary to the male organ during the copulative process; to also sustain the weight of the Uterus; to also afford a passage for the infant at the time of its birth; and also to serve as a passage for the menstrual fluid.

The Uterus, or Womb, is the internal sex organ of the woman which serves to hold the fertilized ovum, or egg, from the time of impregnation, during the period of pregnancy during which the ovum develops into the young child, and until the time of the delivery of the child.

The Uterus is a hollow pear-shaped muscular organ, about three inches in length, nearly an inch thick, and about two inches broad across its upper part, or **fundus**; the lower part, or **cervix**, being much narrower. The **cervix**, or "neck" of the womb, projects into the Vagina, forming the "os uteri," or "mouth of the womb," at that point. The Uterus is composed chiefly of a muscular coat, its walls consisting of strong muscular fibres which contract independently of the will, as do similar muscles in the stomach and bladder. These muscular walls are capable of enormous distention during pregnancy. The muscles of the healthy womb are capable of a tremendous pressure and resistance, and are capable of expelling the child with but slight labor at the time of delivery.

The Uterus is located just behind and slightly above the bladder, and is supported by eight ligaments which, in a healthy condition, hold it firmly and easily in place. Displacements of the Uterus are due to the weakening or relaxing of some or all of these ligaments, generally caused by general weakness or else by excessive physical exercise or labor. The principal **Displacements of the Uterus** are as follows: Prolapsus, or lowering of the womb in the vagina; Antroversion, or the bending forward of the womb; Anteflexion, or the "doubling up" of the womb **forward** on itself; Retroversion, or the bending backward of the womb; and Retroflexion, or the "doubling up" of the womb **backward** on itself. Extreme degrees of the last four mentioned forms of displacement often interfere with impregnation.

The internal surface of the Uterus is lined with mucous membrane thickly studded with minute hairlike cells which manifest continuous motion. This motion, in the lower part of the womb, is in the direction of the fundus or upper part of the womb; in the upper part of the womb, the motion is in the opposite direction; the purpose of these opposing movements being to carry the male elements toward that portion of the womb into which the Fallopian Tubes discharge the products of the Ovaries, as we shall see presently.

The Uterus is supplied with follicles around its neck which secrete a very firm, adhesive mucus substance, which serves as a gate or door across the mouth of the womb during the period of pregnancy, and which also serves to prevent the accidental displacement of the ovum or egg. During and just after menstruation, the Uterus becomes enlarged and more vascular. During pregnancy, it largely increases in weight. After delivery, it resumes its normal size, but the cavity is larger than before conception. In old age, it becomes atrophied and denser in structure.

The Fallopian Tubes are the ducts of the Ovaries, and serve to convey the ova, or eggs, from the Ovaries to the cavity in the Uterus. They are two in number, one on each side, each tube being about four inches in length. They extend from either side of the fundus of the womb, through the broad ligaments which hold them and the Ovaries in position until they communicate with the Ovaries. They are lined with a membrane composed of the same kind of peculiar hair-like cells which are found in the lining of the womb, the purpose in this case being to urge forward the ova or eggs toward the Uterus.

At the ovarian end of the tubes the latter expand into a fringed, trumpet-shaped extremity, the fringe being known as "the fimbria." The tubes are only about one-sixteenth of an inch in diameter, and their small caliber makes it easy for them to clog up as the result of slight inflammation, or to become clogged up or sealed at their mouths or openings, thus causing sterility or inability of the woman to conceive. If the tubes are clogged, or sealed up, it of course is impossible for the ova or eggs to reach the uterus.

The Ovaries are the two oval-shaped bodies lying one on either side of the Uterus. In them the ova, or eggs, are formed. They are each about one and one-half inches long, about one inch wide, and about one-half an inch thick. In addition to their attachment to the broad ligament, they are held in position by folds or ligaments running to the fundus of the Uterus and to the fimbriated extremities of the Fallopian Tubes. The Ovaries are covered by a dense, firm coating which encloses a soft fibrous tissue, abundantly supplied with blood-vessels, which is called the stroma. Imbedded in the mesh-like tissue of the stroma are found numerous small, round, transparent vesicles, in various stages of development, known as the Graafian follicles, which are lined with a layer of peculiar granular cells. These Graafian follicles are the receptacles or sacs which contain the ova, or eggs, which constitute the female reproductive germ. Each vesicle contains a single ovum or egg.

Summary.

From the foregoing, it is seen that we may enumerate the sex organs of the woman as follows, proceeding from the external to the internal organism: First, the Mons Veneris, or prominent eminence above the more important external sex organs; then the Labia Majora, or large outer "lips" or folds, which are plainly discernable to the ordinary view; then the Labia Minora, or smaller inner "lips" or folds, and the Clitoris or small sensitive organ, and the Meatus Urinarius or urinary orifice, all of which are discernable only when the folds of the Labia Majora are parted or opened. Then, proceeding upward and backward from the Vaginal Orifice, we find the Vagina, or channel or canal leading to the Uterus or Womb; then we find the Uterus or Womb at the upper end of the canal or channel of the Vagina. Then extending from either side of the Uterus or Womb we find those two important sets of organs known as the Fallopian Tubes, and the Ovaries, respectively. The Ovaries discharge their ova, or eggs, into the Fallopian Tubes, from whence they are conveyed to the Uterus or Womb, with which the tubes are connected and into which they open at its upper and large end.

The Pelvis is that bony arch in the cavity of which are contained the internal sex organs of the woman. The Pelvis is a bony basin which holds and supports the pelvic organs, and is composed of three important parts, as follows: (1) The Sacrum, consisting of five sections of the vertebral column, or spine, fused together so as to constitute the solid part of the lower spine and the back of the Pelvis; (2) the two Hip-Bones, one on each side of the Pelvis; (3) the Pubic Arch, or the front part of the Pelvis, formed by the junction of the two Hip-Bones in front. Attached to the Hip-Bones are the thighs, and also the large Gluteal Muscles which constitute the buttocks, or "seat."

The Pelvis of the woman is quite different from that of the man. It is shallower and wider, and lighter in structure than that of the male, and the margins of the Hip-Bones are more widely separated, thus making the hips of the woman far more prominent than those of the man. Also, the Sacrum is shorter than that of the man, and the Pubic Arch wider and more rounded than his. This difference in the bony structure is made necessary by the demand for larger space in the female Pelvis required for the purposes of childbirth. These differences are not so perceptible in childhood, but become marked and pronounced at puberty.

LESSON III
PHYSIOLOGY OF THE FEMALE SEX ORGANISM

In the preceding lesson you have been shown "just what" each one of the sex organs of the woman **is**. In the present lesson you will be shown "just what" each of these organs **does**—what its functions and offices are. The preceding lesson dealt with the **anatomy** of these organs; the present lesson will deal with the **physiology** thereof.

Beginning with the Ovaries, the fundamental and basic sex organs of the woman, you will have explained to you the wonderful processes performed by each of these organs in turn.

The Ovaries. The Ovaries in the woman are akin to the testicles in the man. Without the Ovaries there would be no ova or eggs, and without the ova there would be possible no reproductive purposes, and therefore no office for the sex organs at all, for reproduction is the fundamental office, function, and purpose of the entire sexual organism.

In our consideration of the office, purposes, and functions of the Ovaries, however, we must not overlook a certain secondary phase of such functioning. While it is true that the primary purpose of both the testicles of the male, and the Ovaries of the female, is that of providing **seed** from which the offspring of the individual may be produced, it is likewise true that there exists a secondary purpose which may be called the "individual" purpose as contrasted with the "racial" and primary one.

This secondary or "individual" purpose of the Ovaries is that of manufacturing certain secretions which are absorbed by the blood of the woman, and which play an important part in her physical and mental well-being and activities. These secretions begin before puberty in the woman, and continue after her menopause; whereas the manufacture of the ova begins only at puberty, and ceases with the menopause, keeping pace with the manifestation of menstruation in its beginning and its ending.

Nature provides these chemical secretions from the Ovaries for the purpose of giving the woman her characteristic physical form and contour, her form, her breasts, her long hair, her broad pelvis, her soft voice, and other secondary sex characteristics; and also of providing for the normal development of the other sex organs. As a proof of this statement, science shows us that if a woman's ovaries are completely removed there is usually a consequent atrophy or "drying up" of the Uterus and the Vagina, and often even of the Vulva. Moreover, the presence of this internal secretion manifests in arousing and maintaining in the woman her normal sexual desire, and her normal pleasure in the company of her mate; it being noted that if the ovaries are removed, particularly in early life, the woman is apt to lose all sexual desire and normal womanly feeling toward the other sex. And, finally, these secretions make for general physical and mental health and well-being in the woman, and contribute to her vivacity, energy, and activity in all directions. As writers on the subject have well pointed out, this is the reason that capable surgeons usually try to leave at least a portion of the Ovaries when performing an operation for the removal of those organs on account of diseased condition.

The Ovum. The Ovum, or human egg, is a small spherical body, measuring from one two-hundred-and-fortieth to one one-hundred-and-twentieth of an inch in diameter. It has a colorless transparent envelope, the latter enclosing the yolk which consists of granules or globules of various sizes embedded in a viscid fluid. In the center of the yolk is found a very small vesicular body consisting of a tenuous transparent membrane, which is known as "the germinal vesicle;" this, in turn, contains a very tiny granular structure, opaque, of yellow color, known as "the germinal spot."

When the time is reached in which the ovum or egg is to be discharged, the Graafian follicle becomes enlarged by reason of the accumulation of the fluids in its interior, and exerts such a steady and increasing pressure from within, outward, that the surrounding tissue yields to it, and it finally protrudes from the Ovary, from whence it is then expelled with a gush, owing to the elasticity and reaction of the neighboring tissues.

Following this rupture there occurs an abundant hemorrhage from the vesicles of the follicle, the cavity being filled with blood, which then coagulates and is retained in the Graafian follicle. The formation and development of the Graafian follicle begins at puberty and continues until the menopause or "change of life" of the woman. Many follicles are produced, but many do not produce ova, and so gradually atrophy. The ripening and discharge of the eggs produce a peculiar condition of congestion of the entire female sexual organism, including the Fallopian Tubes, the Uterus, the Vagina, and even of the Vulva, which results in a condition of Sexual Excitement. Among the lower animals the female will allow the male to approach her for copulation only at this period, this being the time when the egg is ready for fertilization.

When the female infant is born, her Ovaries contain the germs of about 100,000 ova. The greater portion of these, however, disappear, until at the time of her puberty the number of germs of ova contains only about 30,000 ova. This number is far more than the woman will ever need, and is Nature's provision against diseased portions of the Ovaries, accidents, etc. Only one ovum ripens and matures each month from puberty until menopause, so that the woman really requires only about 300 to 350 ova on the average. This liberality on the part of Nature, however, does not begin to approach her lavishness in the case of seed of the male, for in his case while only one spermatozoon is required to fertilize an ovum (and in fact only one is permitted to do so), we find that in each normal act of ejaculation of semen by the male over 250,000 spermatozoa are projected.

The ripening and discharge of the egg from the Ovaries, and the consequent congestion above referred to, accompanied by what is called Menstruation, occurs regularly each lunar month (28 days). What is called Ovulation consists of the monthly maturing and expulsion of the ripe ovum or egg, while Menstruation (as we shall see later on) consists of the monthly discharge of blood and mucus from the inner surface of the Uterus; the two processes occur in connection with each other, yet neither can be considered as the cause of the other.

Menstruation. It may be well to call your attention at this point to the process known as Menstruation, or "the monthly flow," or "the courses" of women. Menstruation is the monthly flow of bloody fluid which occurs in all healthy (non-pregnant) women from puberty to the menopause or "change of life."

By "**Puberty**" is meant the age at which a woman begins her period of possible child-bearing experience. In temperate climates the average age of puberty is about fourteen years, while in tropical countries it is often a year or so earlier, and in arctic countries a year or so later. The time, however, depends materially upon the temperament, race, hygiene, and general environment of the individual girl. At this period the girl gradually changes into the young woman. Her figure changes, her bust develops, her hips broaden, and her mental and emotional nature undergoes a change. Also the menstrual flow begins to manifest at this time; at first scanty and irregular, but gradually changing into the characteristic flow each month.

At the period of puberty, the girl undergoes marked emotional changes. She becomes very "emotional" as a rule, and quite "sensitive." She becomes filled with strange, unaccountable longings, ideas, and "notions." She usually manifests a great emotional interest in her girl friends, and often manifests marked jealousy in connection with these friendships. The girl is apt to indulge in day-dreaming at this period, and becomes quite romantic and "flighty." She devours love stories, and delights in imagining herself as the heroine of similar adventures. The period from the beginning of puberty to that of the attainment of full sexual maturity is known as the period of "adolescence," and generally extends to about the age of eighteen in the case of girls.

By the **Menopause** is meant that period of the woman's "change of life," the average time of which is about the age of forty-five years, although this varies greatly in different individuals. As a rule, it is held that the period of the woman's child-bearing possibility extends over an average period of thirty years. At the Menopause the woman's reproductive activity declines and finally ends. The Ovaries diminish in size, the Graafian follicles cease to form and develop; the Fallopian Tubes atrophy; and there occur other physical, mental, and emotional changes in the woman. While the age of forty-five is held to be the average age at which the Menopause occurs in women, still it is not at all uncommon to find women who menstruate regularly up to the age of fifty, or fifty-two, or even fifty-five, while a large number of women menstruate regularly at the age of forty-eight.

Some women undergo little or no physical or emotional disturbance at the time of the Menopause. In such cases their periods become more or less irregular, with extending intervals between periods; the flow becomes more and more scanty; then several periods are skipped altogether; and finally the periods cease entirely. Other women, however, experience more or less physical disturbance during the years of the "change." They sometimes experience loss of appetite, or a capricious appetite, headaches, loss of weight, or else a sudden taking on of fatty tissue. They often become quite irritable and "notiony," and often become quarrelsome and pugnacious, and in some cases manifest unreasonable jealousy. But, in the opinion of many of the best authorities, much of this trouble comes from the mental expectancy of them by the woman, resulting from the notion that a woman must have these things happen to her. The power of the mind over the body is now well known, and we have here another instance of its effect. The remedy is obvious.

Another matter which disturbs the woman at this time, in many cases, is the common belief that after "the change" she will lose all of her sex attractiveness, and her sexual feelings, etc. This is a grave error, for the experience of all observing physicians is that no such results follow this period of the woman's life. Many women become even more attractive to the other sex after this time, by reason of acquiring a certain maturity and "ripeness" which proves very attractive to many men—often to young men as well as older ones. Moreover, the sexual desires do not cease with the cessation of the reproductive functions. On the contrary, it often happens that such emotions and desires are increased in the woman at, and after, this time of her life. So true is this that this period has been called "The Dangerous Age" for women, and the experience of many a woman of forty-five to fifty will corroborate this statement. The woman at this time should beware of contracting unwise love affairs and entanglements, and of yielding to impulses toward men other than her mate. A word to the wise should be sufficient in this case.

To return to the main subject of Menstruation, it may be said that the monthly flow, when once established, occurs at intervals of every twenty-eight days, on the average, although in some individual cases it occurs as often as every twenty-one days, while in others it occurs as seldom as once in every six weeks, all without exceeding the bounds of normal functioning. Menstruation ceases temporarily during pregnancy, in normal cases, and often also ceases during the period of lactation or nursing. The menstrual period lasts on an average for four or five days, the flow increasing for the first half of the period, and decreasing during the last half. At the beginning of the period there is often manifested a general congestion of all of the sexual organs of the woman, and often of the breasts as well. There is also usually found a sense of physical discomfort, from which more or less irritable feeling arises. In rare cases there are found severe cramps and pains, and in some cases the woman finds it necessary to call in medical aid, or to go to bed, or both. In such cases a cure is often worked by improving the general health, and by observing common sense hygienic rules.

Menstruation is caused by a hypertrophy of the mucus membrane of inner surface of the Uterus, which is followed by a shedding of the hypertrophied membrane. This leaves exposed the underlying vessels, which bleed. New mucus membrane is formed after the period. The menstrual flow consists of a thin, bloody fluid, having peculiar odor, in which is combined blood, thin skin, and mucus membrane, and also mucus from the Uterus and the Vagina, the blood being light in consistency and not clotted.

During the menstrual period the ovum, or egg, is discharged, and enters the Uterus, as we shall see presently.

The Life-History of the Ovum. The physiology of the remaining sexual organs of the woman may perhaps best be studied by considering the story of the Life-History of the Ovum, or human egg, for the functions of such organs are concerned with such life-history of the egg, and really exist merely to create such a history, or rather, to produce the process which constitutes the basis of such history.

The ovum, or egg, when discharged from the ovary, is at first surrounded by a few cells which serve as nourishment, but which soon disappear. It enters the Fallopian Tube and begins its journey toward the Uterus, being urged on its way by the constant movement of the lining-cells of the interior of the tube, in the direction of the Uterus. Certain changes in structure occur. Its passage to the Uterus may be interrupted, and the ovum lost and finally cast off. But the ovum that is successful finally arrives at the Uterus where it awaits impregnation or fertilization by the spermatozoon of the male.

If copulation occurs within a reasonable time after the arrival of the ovum, it is impregnated or fertilized. Fecundation results and conception ensues, the ovum then remaining attached to the walls of the Uterus, and in time develops into the foetus. If, however, the ovum is not impregnated, because of absence of copulation or from other causes, it gradually loses its vitality, and is finally cast off with the several uterine secretions.

It should be explained here that the "spermatozoon" of the male (the plural of the term is "spermatozoa") is the male generative "seed." The sperum, semen, or seminal fluid of the male is filled with hundreds of thousands of spermatozoa. Each spermatozoon is a minute living, moving creature, resembling a microscopic tadpole. It has a head, a rod-like body, and a thin hair-like tail, the latter being kept in constant motion from side to side, by means of which the tiny creature is enabled to travel rapidly from one point to another. The human spermatozoon measures about one six-hundredth of an inch in length. It is composed of protoplasm, the substance of which all living creatures are composed. The spermatozoa are believed to be developed from a parent sperm-cell, by the process of segmentation or subdivision, which process is common to all cell-life. The numerous spermatozoa dwell in a gelatinous substance, which, mingling with the other fluidic secretions of the glands of the male, constitutes the male seminal fluid, sperm, or semen, which is ejaculated by the male during the process of copulation.

Fecundation (i. e. fertilization, impregnation; the process by which the male reproductive element is brought in contact with the female ovum or egg) is brought about by the blending of the male reproductive element (or spermatozoon) with the female reproductive element (or ovum, or egg). This blending is of course accomplished by the bringing together in mutual contact the two reproductive elements just mentioned. The sexual act which results in this "bringing together" of the two elements is known as "copulation," or "coition." In copulation or coition the seminal fluid of the male, containing an enormous number of spermatozoa, is ejaculated from the male intromittent organ into the receptive canal or channel of the female (the Vagina), and in this way finally comes into actual contact with the female ovum or egg which is awaiting it in the Uterus of the female.

The spermatozoa (in the process of copulation) are deposited in the Vagina of the female, usually at its upper end, but sometimes in the lower portion; and in rare and peculiar cases even at or about the Vaginal Orifice or outer vaginal opening. In either case they travel up the remaining portion of the Vagina and finally enter the Uterus or womb. The spermatozoa possess wonderful vitality and power of locomotion. There are cases recorded in which the spermatozoa deposited on or about the outer female genitals have managed to travel inward and upward until they have finally reached the Uterus, where conception has resulted. Such cases, of course, are rare, but they exist, well authenticated and accepted by medical science as facts.

It must not be supposed, however, that the impregnation of the ovum occurs only in the womb proper. Cases are known in which the spermatozoa have traveled along the Fallopian Tubes and impregnated the ovum there; and in very rare cases the spermatozoon seems to have penetrated even to the Ovary itself, and there impregnated the ovum on the surface of the Ovary. Some excellent authorities, in fact, insist that all normal impregnation occurs at the end of the Fallopian Tube—the point of its entrance into the upper part of the womb, rather than in the body of the womb, or at its mouth, as the older authorities taught. But wherever the actual contact of spermatozoon and ovum occurs, the blending of the elements is performed and fertilization, impregnation, or fecundation is accomplished.

As a result of copulation, then, the spermatozoon (or a number of spermatozoa) comes in contact with the female ovum or egg. Then one or more of them, by means of a furious lashing of the tiny tail, manages to penetrate the outer covering of the ovum, and enters the space between the outer covering and the real body of the egg. Several spermatozoa may effect an entrance into this outer space, **but only one is permitted to enter the real body of the egg**. [Twins are produced by the impregnation of two ova by two spermatozoa, at the same time. The presence of the two ova at the same time is unusual]. The moment that the real body of the ovum is penetrated by the successful spermatozoon, a tough covering or thick membrane forms around the ovum and thus prevents the entrance of other spermatozoa. The successful spermatozoon then loses its tail, and the remaining head and body become what is known as "the male pronucleus."

The authorities are uncertain as to the exact nature of the change which occurs when the ovum is penetrated by the spermatozoon. The outward manifestations of the change and transformation arising from the blending of the male and female elements are of course well known, but the "life process" eludes the power of the microscope. When Nature forms the thick membranous coating over the impregnated ovum, she draws the veil over one of her most important secrets. The first segmentation-nucleus having been formed by the blending and forging together of the male and female pronuclei, the process of segmentation begins.

Segmentation proceeds as follows: the impregnated egg splits into halves, forming two joined cells; then into quarters, forming four joined cells; then into sixteenths, then into thirty-seconds, sixty-fourths, and so on, until the ovum consists of a combined mass of very minute granular-like cells, the whole resembling a mulberry. The segmentation of the nucleus precedes and then continues with the segmentation of the yolk. After the egg has been divided into a great number of these cells, the latter begin a centrifugal action resulting in the formation of a complete inner lining of closely packed cells, with a central cavity filled with the yolk liquid.

In the meantime, the Uterus has been prepared for the reception of the impregnated and transformed ovum. A thick, spongy, juicy, mucus membrane forms, into which the changing ovum passes and attaches itself; the mucus membrane soon enveloping it and shutting it off from the rest of the Uterus. There now appears at one point on the ovum an opaque streak, which is called "the primitive trace" of the embryo—the first beginning of the young living creature. The "primitive trace" then grows in length and breadth. At this point we must leave the history of the ovum, or human egg, for the present; its further development will be related in the succeeding lesson, the subject of which is "Gestation."

LESSON IV
GESTATION OR PREGNANCY

Gestation is "the act of carrying young in the Uterus, from the time of conception to that of parturition." Conception occurs at the moment of the impregnation of the ovum; parturition is the act of delivery, or childbirth. Pregnancy is "the state of being with child." The terms "period of gestation," and "period of pregnancy," respectively, are employed by medical authorities to designate the time during which the mother carries the young within her own body—from the moment of the impregnation of the ovum until the moment of the final delivery of the child into the outer world.

The term of pregnancy in woman continues for over nine calendar months (or ten lunar months)—from about 275 to 280 days, though in exceptional cases it may be terminated in seven calendar months, or on the other hand may continue for ten calendar months. The usual method is to figure 280 days from the **first day** of the **last menstruation**. A simple method of calculating the probable date of delivery is as follows: **Count back three months, and then add seven days, and you will have the date of probable delivery.** Example: A woman's **first day of last menstruation** is March 28. Counting back three months gives us December 28; and adding seven days to this gives us January 4, as the date of probable delivery. There will always be a possible margin of a few days before or after the ascertained probable date—but the delivery will very closely approximate said date. Ignore the shortage of days of February in this calculation, the same being covered by the general margin allowed.

Development of the Impregnated Ovum. In the preceding lesson we terminated our consideration of the impregnated ovum at the point at which, after the process of segmentation, the "primitive trace" had appeared. This primitive trace appears as an opaque streak, or straight line, formed of an aggregation of cells of a distinctive quality. This delicate "trace" or "streak" is the first indication of the form of the coming child. It is the basis, pattern, or mould, in or around which the spinal column is to be formed, and around which the entire young body is to be developed by the wonderful and intricate processes of dividing and reduplication, and the folding and combination of cells. From one end of this "trace" develops the head; from the other end develops the lower end of the spine. At a later stage there appear tiny "buds" in the positions at which the arms and legs should be; these gradually develop, and their ends split into tiny fingers and toes, and finally are transformed into perfect little arms and legs, miniatures of those of the adult human being.

The term "the embryo" is employed to designate the developing young creature in the earlier stages of its development, particularly before the end of the third month of its existence. After the end of the third month the embryo is called "the fetus." In the short space of 280 days the young creature evolves and develops from a single simple cell into a complex organism—a perfect miniature human being. Nature works a wonderful miracle here, and yet so common is it that we take it all as a matter of course, and lose sight of the miracle. From the most simple forms are formed in the developing creature the most complex organs and parts. The heart is formed from a tiny straight line of cells, by enlargement and partition. The stomach and intestines, likewise, develop from a tiny straight line of cells arranged as a tiny tube—the stomach is formed by dilation of one part of the tube, while the large intestine experiences a similar though lesser distention and a greater growth in length; the smaller intestines being formed by growth in length and circumference. The other organs evolve from similar simple beginnings.

The embryo is nourished during its earlier stages by means of the "yolk sack," or "umbilical vesicle," which is outside the body of the embryo, being joined to it by means of the umbilical duct. This yolk sack (originally formed by a "drawing together" in the ovum, which thus separates itself into two portions or areas) is an important feature of the life of the embryo, as it nourishes and sustains it in its earlier stages. Blood vessels form in this yolk sack, and after a time its fluid is absorbed, and after the third month the sack gradually disappears.

After the passing away of the yolk sack, the embryo is nourished and sustained by the "allantois," another peculiar sack which is formed. This sack readily becomes filled with blood-vessels, and serves to nourish the embryo by sustenance obtained from the body of the mother through the walls of the Uterus, a direct communication with the blood-vessels of the mother thus being secured. The blood in the embryo, and that in the mother, come into close contact, thus allowing the embryo to be nourished by the blood of the mother. After a time, in turn, the allantois diminishes and dwindles away, its offices being taken up and performed by the "placenta" or "afterbirth."

The Placenta or Afterbirth. The Placenta, or afterbirth, is a round, flat substance or organ, contained within the Uterus, by which communication and connection is established and maintained between the fetus and the mother, by means of the umbillical cord. It is a flat, circular mass, about seven inches in diameter, and weighing about sixteen ounces. It is attached to the sides of the Uterus of the mother during the period of gestation, and is expelled from the body of the mother, as "the afterbirth," after the birth of the child.

Let us pause a moment, and reconsider the several steps in Nature's plan for nourishing the embryo and fetus. In the first place, as we have seen, there is the yolk sack or umbillical vesicle, filled with a fluid which nourishes the embryo. This gradually disappears in time, and is replaced by the "allantois" which by connection with the walls of the Uterus is enabled to nourish the fetus from and by the blood of the mother. For a short time, however, the embryo is nourished by both the yolk sack and the allantois. Then the allantois assumes the entire task, and the yolk sack passes away. Then, later, the placenta replaces the allantois, and the latter passes away as did its predecessor. The placenta works along the same general lines as the allantois, but is a far more complex way and with a much higher degree of efficiency, as we shall see presently.

The placenta is connected with the body of the fetus by what is known as "the umbillical cord." The "umbillicus" or "navel" in the human being marks the place at which the umbillical cord entered the body of the fetus, from which it was severed after the birth of the child. The purpose of the umbillical cord is to contain and support the umbillical arteries and veins through which the fetus obtains nourishment from the placental substance, and through which the return blood flows. The rich red arterial blood is carried from the placenta to the fetus, and is then distributed over the body of the fetus, nourishing and building it up; the dark venous blood, laden with the waste products of the body of the fetus, is carried back to the placenta, there to be repurified and rendered again rich and nourishing.

The story of the circulation of the blood of the fetus is most interesting. Although the fetal blood is derived from that of the mother, as we have said, yet the maternal blood does not pass directly from the circulatory system of the mother into that of the fetus; nor does the blood of the fetus return directly into the circulatory system of the mother. In fact, the fetal blood never comes in direct contact with that of the mother, or vice versa. The fetus has an independent circulatory system of its own, and yet, at the same time, from the moment of the placental connection until the moment of childbirth, all its nourishment is derived from its mother.

The secret of the above paradoxical statement is made apparent when we understand the meaning of the scientific term "osmosis." Osmosis is "the passage of a fluid through a membrane"; it is a chemical process, caused by the chemical affinity between two liquids or gases separated one from the other by a porous diaphragm or substance. In the process of osmosis in the case before us, the fetal blood takes up nourishing substances and oxygen from the blood of the mother, and passes on to the latter the waste products of the fetal system, by means of passing these substances through the thin porous membranes which separate the two independent systems of blood vessels, i. e., the system of the fetus, and that of the mother. Before birth, in fact, the fetus has its blood nourished and oxygenated by means of the food partaken of by its mother, and the oxygen taken in by the mother in her breathing. After its birth, the infant eats and breathes for itself, and thus nourishes its blood supply directly, instead of receiving it indirectly from the mother.

The Placenta begins to be formed about the third month of gestation, and continues to develop steadily from that time. At the time of the delivery of the child the Placenta covers nearly or quite one-third of the inner space of the distended Uterus of the mother. The total "afterbirth" consists of the Placenta, the umbillical cord, and the remaining membranes of the ovum, all of which are expelled after the birth of the child.

The Amnion. An important appendage contained in the Uterus in connection with the developing fetus is that known as "The Amnion." This is an inner sack which forms within the womb, and which serves to enclose the fetus, and also to sheath the umbillical cord. The Amnion encloses the embryo very snugly during the early stages of its development, but it gradually becomes distended with a pale watery fluid, known as "the amniotic fluid," the purpose of which is to "float" the fetus and to give it mechanical support on all sides. This fluid is composed of water carrying in solution small quantities of albumin, urea, and salt.

Sex in the Embryo and Fetus. It is impossible to determine the sex of the embryo during its early stages. During the fourth week the first traces of the sexual glands appear, but not until the fifth week can the sex be determined even by the microscope. If the embryo is to become a male, certain ducts are transformed into convoluted tubules, and each is attached to the testes which have been formed from the genital nucleus. If the embryo is to become a female, the ducts join to form the uterus and vagina, other portions being transformed into the fallopian tubes and connecting with the ovaries which have been formed otherwise. The outer genitals appear in the early stages of the embryo, but there is no apparent distinction between the sexes, the external organs being the same in all cases, and consisting of a small tubular organ with a small lateral fold of skin on either side. Later, in the male, a groove appears on the under side of this primitive organ, thus forming the urethra, the scrotum being formed from the folded skin at the side. In the female, the primitive organ ceases to develop as in the male, and thus becomes proportionately smaller, and evolves into the clitoris of the female; the two lateral folds, on each side, being transformed into the labia majora, or "outer lips" of the female external genitals.

Position of the Fetus. During the period of gestation the fetus lies "curled up" in the bag of the amnion. The head is usually relaxed and inclined forward, the chin resting on the breast; the feet are bent up in front of the legs, the legs bent up on the thighs, the knees separated from each other, but the heels almost touching on the back of the thighs; the arms bent forward and the hands placed between them as though to receive the chin between them. The folded-up fetus forms an oval, the longest diameter of which is about eleven inches at its greatest stage of growth. Nature here shows a wonderful ability to pack the fetus into as little space as possible, and in such a position as to protect it from injury, and to discommode the mother as little as possible.

The following interesting statement made by Helen Idleson, M. D., in a European medical journal several years ago, gives a very clear idea, expressed in popular terms, of the appearance and characteristics of the embryo or fetus in the various stages of its development:

"The growth of the embryo after fecundation is very rapid. On the **tenth day** it has the appearance of a semi-transparent grayish flake. On the **twelfth day** it is nearly the size of a pea, filled with fluid, in the middle of which is an opaque spot, presenting the first appearance of an embryo, which may be clearly seen as an oblong or curved body, and is plainly visible to the naked eye on the fourteenth day. The **twenty-first day** the embryo resembles an ant or a lettuce seed. Many of its parts now begin to show themselves, especially the cartilaginous beginnings of the spinal column, the heart, etc. The **thirtieth day** the embryo is as large as a horse-fly, and resembles a worm, bent together. There are as yet no limbs, and the head is larger than the rest of the body. When stretched out it is nearly half an inch long. Toward the fifth week the heart increases greatly in proportion to the remainder of the body, and the rudimentary eyes are indicated by two black spots toward the sides, and the heart exhibits its external form, bearing a close resemblance to that in an adult. In the **seventh week**, bone begins to form in the lower jaw and clavicle. Narrow streaks on each side of the vertebral column show the beginning of the ribs. The heart is perfecting its form, the brain enlarging, and the eyes and ears growing more perfect, and the limbs sprouting from the body. The lungs are mere sacks, and the trachea is a delicate thread, but the liver is very large. In the seventh week are formed the renal capsules and kidneys.

"At **two months**, the forearm and hand can be distinguished, but not the arm; the hand is larger than the forearm, but it is not supplied with fingers. The distinction of sex is yet difficult. The eyes are prominent. The nose forms an obtuse eminence. The nostrils are rounded and separated. The mouth is gaping, and the epidermis can be distinguished from the true skin. The embryo is from one-half to two inches long, the head forming more than one-third of the whole. At the end of **three months**, the eyelids are distinct but shut; the lips are drawn together; the forehead and nose are clearly traceable, and the organs of generation prominent. The heart beats with force; the larger vessels carry red blood; the fingers and toes are well defined, and the muscles begin to be developed.

"At the **fourth month**, the embryo takes the name of 'fetus.' The body is six to eight inches in length. The skin has a rosy color, and the muscles produce a sensible motion. A fetus born at this time might live several hours. At **five months** the length of the body is from eight to ten inches. At **six months**, the length is twelve and one-half inches. The hair appears on the head, the eyes closed, the eyelids somewhat thicker, and their margins, as well as their eyebrows, are studded with very delicate hairs. At **seven months**, every part has been increased in volume and perfection; the bony system is nearly complete; length, twelve to fourteen inches. If born at this period, the fetus is able to breathe, cry and nurse, and may live if properly cared for.

"At **eight months**, the fetus seems to grow rather in length than in thickness; it is only sixteen to eighteen inches long, and yet weighs from four to five pounds. The skin is very red, and covered with down and a considerable quantity of sebaceous matter. The lower jaw, which at first was very short, is now as long as the upper one. Finally, at term, **nine months**, the fetus is about nineteen to twenty-three inches long, and weighs from six to eight pounds. The red blood circulates in the capillaries, and the skin performs the functions of perspiration; the nails are fully developed."

Another writer says: "There is a superstition that a child born at eight months is not as liable to live as if born at seven months; indeed, many suppose that an eight months' child never survives. Facts do not prove this idea to be correct. Personally, I have known several eight months' babies to live and do well, and I believe that their chance of life is much greater than if born at seven months."

Children born in the seventh month of gestation are capable of living, though great care is required to rear them for the first few months after birth. The "incubators" now so common in large cities have greatly increased the chances of the "seven months' child," and, for that matter, of those born even earlier. There are a number of cases of record where children have been born after six months of gestation, and a few even before the six months, but these cases are rare and unusual, and such children usually die soon after birth.

The following table, given by a good authority, shows the average length and weight of the human embryo and fetus:

Age.	Length in inches.	Weight.
2 weeks	0.1	Not given
3 weeks	0.2	3 grains
4 weeks	0.3	Not given
5 weeks	0.5	Not given
6 weeks	0.7	Not given
7 weeks	0.9	Not given
8 weeks	1.5	4 drachms
3 months	3.0	2 ounces
4 months	6.0	5 ounces
5 months	9.0	10 ounces
6 months	12.0	1 pound
7 months	15.0	3 pounds
8 months	17.0	5 pounds
9 months	20.0	6 to 9 pounds

Professor Clark holds that if at birth the infant weighs less than 5 pounds, it rarely thrives, though the records show that many infants weighing much less than this have lived and thrived. In very rare cases, infants have been known to weigh no more than one pound at birth, and to have still survived and thrived. And, on the other hand, many cases are known where infants were born, and thrived, who weighed more than twice the average weight. So, at the last, it is difficult to lay down hard and fast rules in the case.

Delivery. At the termination of the period of gestation, the child is born into the world, and, instead of depending upon the blood of the mother for nourishment and oxygen, it begins to ingest its own food, to eliminate its own waste matter through the regular channels of the body, and to use its own lungs for the purpose of obtaining oxygen for its blood and to burn up the waste products in the lungs.

The process of bringing a child into the world is called "parturition." The fetus is expelled from the body of the mother by the contraction of the muscles of and around the Uterus, and also by the contraction of the abdominal walls. In the early stages of labor, the uterine muscles are brought into play; but when the fetus enters into the vaginal passage the abdominal muscles manifest their energy. The uterine and abdominal muscular movements are purely involuntary, although the mother may aid in the delivery by voluntary muscular movements. The involuntary muscular movements are due to the reflex action originating, probably, in a part of the spinal cord.

The uterine contractions are rhythmical, and have been compared to the contraction of the muscles of the heart. Each "labor pain" begins with a minimum of contraction, the activity increasing until a maximum is reached, when it gradually decreases, only to be followed a little later by a new contraction. When the fetus is finally expelled from the Uterus (followed later by the placenta or "afterbirth") that organ begins a gradual contraction to its normal size, shape, and condition, the restorative process usually lasting over several weeks.

The Physical Signs of Pregnancy. The physical signs of pregnancy in the case of women of normal health are as follows:

(1) Cessation of the menses, or menstruation. While it is true that a non-pregnant woman may occasionally pass over a menstrual period, yet as a general rule the complete cessation of a period by a married woman, particularly when the woman has previously been regular in this respect, may be considered a probable indication of pregnancy; and when the second period has been passed the probability merges almost into a certainty. An examination by a competent physician will set all doubts at rest.

(2) Enlargement of the breasts. This indication usually manifests itself in about six or eight weeks after conception. This enlargement is usually preceded by a sensation of tingling and throbbing. The enlargement is manifested in the form of a rather hard and knotty increase, differing from the ordinary fatty increase; the lobules, arranged regularly around the nipple, are plainly distinguishable beneath the skin by means of the touch of the fingers.

(3) Darkening of the areolar tissue surrounding the nipple. In the unimpregnated condition this tissue is of a pinkish shade; but after impregnation the shade grows darker and the circle increases in size. However, when the woman bears several children in somewhat rapid succession, this dark color may become permanent and accordingly ceases to be an indication.

(4) Enlargement of the abdomen. This indication manifests itself about the second month, at which time the Uterus begins to elevate the intestines by rising up from the pelvis. In the fourth month the Uterus has risen so far out of the pelvis that it assumes the form and appearance of a hard round tumor. The entire abdomen then begins to enlarge. The Uterus causes an enlargement in the region of the navel at the sixth month, and the region of the diaphragm at the ninth month.

(5) Quickening, or "signs of life." This indication manifests first from the fourth month to the fifth—at about the exact half of the entire period of gestation. At this time, and afterward, the movements of the embryo are plainly discernable to the mother.

The Disorders of Pregnancy. There are a number of physical disorders usually accompanying pregnancy, some of which are trifling, but some of which require the advice of a competent physician. The best plan is for the woman to consult a physician shortly after she discovers herself to be pregnant, and thereafter to visit him occasionally for advice during the period of gestation. The too common plan of postponing the call upon the physician until the eighth or ninth month is not a wise one, for in many cases the advice of a competent physician at an earlier stage of the pregnancy will obviate serious complications. The call upon the physician should usually be made not later than the third or fourth month, and positively not delayed longer than the fifth month. The physician should make an examination to ascertain whether the child is in the normal position in the Uterus, and should also examine the urine each month to ascertain whether the kidneys are functioning normally.

What is called "morning sickness" is one of the most common of the disorders of pregnancy. It is marked by nausea or vomiting, or both, early in the morning, usually shortly after arising. Some women have at least faint symptoms of this disorder from the very beginning of conception, but usually it does not manifest until the third, fourth, or fifth week of pregnancy. It usually ceases at the end of the third or fourth month. Except in very severe cases, in which the physician should be consulted, the disorder is not serious, and requires but a little common-sense treatment, and rational habits of living. An authority says: "Eat of some fruit that best agrees with palate or stomach; drink hot water; eat nothing until a real hunger demands food. Where nausea occurs after eating, a tart apple or orange is good." Another authority says: "Let women suffering from morning sickness try acid fruit—apples, oranges, or even lemons, if their sourness is not unpleasant. If a single orange or apple after each meal does not suffice, let them try two; let them eat ten if that number is necessary to conquer the distress. The principle is a correct one, and the relief certain. Let fruit be eaten at all hours of the day—before meals and after, on going to bed at night and at getting up in the morning. If berries are in season, let them be eaten in the natural state—that is, without sugar. If the sickness still continues, omit a meal now and then, and substitute fruit in its stead. By persistence in this course, not only will nausea be conquered, but an easy confinement guaranteed."

The pregnant woman often develops a capricious appetite. This disorder may manifest in one or more of several forms, as for instance: the woman may lose her appetite, and take but little food; or she may develop an abnormally large appetite, and eat much more than is necessary; or she may take a dislike to certain kinds of food—many women have an aversion toward meat during pregnancy; or she may have a "craving" for certain articles of food, sometimes for kinds of food not liked at other times, such as sour pickles, sour cabbage, etc. A little common sense, and the presence of attractive articles of fruits, etc., will do much to relieve these troubles; in extreme cases the physician's advice will help.

The pregnant woman should have her teeth put in good order as soon as possible, as troubles with teeth sometimes manifest themselves during pregnancy, and give much trouble and annoyance. Difficulty in urination, constipation, piles, irritation or itching of the genital organs, varicose veins, liver spots, and similar disorders, which are sometimes manifest during pregnancy, in some form or degree, should receive the attention and care of a competent physician.

The following general advice from a competent authority is worthy of being followed: "If everything is satisfactory, if there is no severe vomiting, kidney trouble, etc., the usual mixed diet may continue. The only changes I would make are the following: Drink plenty of hot water during the entire time of pregnancy: a glass or two in the morning, two or three glasses in the afternoon, the same at night. From six to twelve glasses may be consumed. Also plenty of milk, buttermilk and fermented milk. Plenty of fruit and vegetables. Meat only once a day. For the tendency to constipation, whole wheat bread, rye bread, bread baked of bran, or bran with cream. As to exercise, either extreme must be avoided. Some women think that as soon as they become pregnant, they must not move a muscle; they are to be put in a glass case, and kept there until the date of delivery. Other women, on the other hand, of the ultra-modern type, indulge in strenuous exercise, and go out on long fatiguing walks up to the last day. Either extreme is injurious. The right way is moderate exercise, and short, non-fatiguing walks. Bathing may be kept up to the day of the delivery. But warm baths, particularly during the last two or three months, are preferable to cold baths."

Childbirth. The first indication of approaching delivery of the child is that of the descent of the child into the pelvis of the mother, from its former position up near the diaphragm. When this occurs, the mother usually experiences a feeling of relief, and a greater ease in breathing because of the relaxation of the former pressure on the diaphragm. Sometimes this occurs several days preceding delivery, while in other cases it occurs only a few hours before delivery. There usually occurs about the same time a slight discharge of mucus tinged with blood. The latter is called "the show," and is caused by the unsealing of the mouth of the womb, and indicates that the Uterus is preparing to discharge its contents.

Labor, in childbirth, consists of three stages. In the first stage, the Uterus alone contracts, and the mouth of the womb dilates; in the second stage, the abdominal muscles assist the Uterus in expelling the child; in the third stage, the Placenta (afterbirth) and membranes are expelled.

After the delivery of the child, and after the pulsation in the umbillical cord has ceased (usually from ten to thirty minutes after delivery), the umbillical cord is severed and tied by the physician. In natural labor, the expulsion of the afterbirth occurs from within a few minutes to an hour after the delivery of the child. Nature is sometimes slow in expelling the afterbirth, but caution should be exercised in the matter of using force to assist Nature in this matter, for injury to the Uterus has often resulted from malpractice in such a case. The afterbirth is not firmly attached to the womb, but is like the peel of an orange which Nature sloughs off in due time.

LESSON V
GENERAL ADVICE TO WOMEN ON SEX SUBJECTS

In this lesson the writer seeks to direct the attention of his women readers to certain subjects upon which the average woman is not well informed, and upon which she usually requires sound, sane, clean, frank information. In many cases women hesitate to ask even their family physicians for such information, and, although there is no rational reason for it, they even shrink from consulting better informed and capable women concerning these subjects.

Sexual Feeling. Owing to erroneous teachings, and irrational prejudices arising from ancient distorted and perverted ideals of sex, many women have grown to maturity under the erroneous belief that it is a sign of immorality, or at least low ideals and depraved nature, for a woman to experience sexual emotions or feelings, wishes or desires. So true is this that even many married women seek to withhold from their husbands the knowledge that any sexual feeling is experienced by the wife.

Such a belief is of course absurd. It is as natural for a woman to experience normal sexual feeling as it is for her to experience any other feeling aroused by natural instincts and organism. Without such instinct and the feelings arising therefrom, there would be no mating or marriage, and no perpetuation of the race. The woman experiencing such feelings should not allow herself to imagine that she is depraved or perverted, or immoral in thought and feeling. Incredible as it may appear to a normal, healthy-minded man, it is true that thousands of young women have lost self-respect, and have lapsed into a morbid state of mind, because of the occasional manifestation of their normal sexual feeling.

This does not, of course, mean that the woman must necessarily manifest into action the feeling experienced by her. On the contrary, she must acquire self-mastery and self-control, just as she must in other phases of her life. It may help some women of this kind to realize that the sex feeling and impulses, arising unbidden (and often unwelcomed) from the depths of their subconscious mentality, are essentially **creative** impulses. If the woman be unmarried, or if married and placed under conditions in which the marital relation with the husband is impossible or undesirable, then she can **transmute** this creative energy in some form of creative work—in work which leads to the creation, manufacture, building-up, or composing something. There is a hint here which will prove a great blessing to the woman who will understand and apply the principle suggested—for many other women have found it so.

As for the married woman, there is no reason whatsoever why she should seek to withhold from her husband the knowledge that she is possessed of normal, natural, healthy sexual feeling. In fact, the withholding of such information, and the concealment and deception arising therefrom, has often done much to bring marital inharmony between husband and wife. If there is any deception to be practiced in the marital association of husband and wife, it should rather be in the opposite direction, i. e., in the direction of pretending the emotional feeling when it exists only partially or is absent. The last matter, however, is one for the exercise of the judgment and conviction of each individual woman; but the first mentioned admonition is one which should be observed, as it is based on honesty, truth, and good judgment as well.

Alcohol and Sexuality. It needs no extended argument to convince the average person that an individual will do things when under the influence of drink that he or she would not do when perfectly sober. It is an old saying that "When the wine is in, the wits are out." But there is a deeper connection and relation between alcoholic drink and sexual indiscretions than is usually realized by the average person. Besides the commonly known weakening of will-power and self-control arising from the influence of strong drink, there are certain influences concerning the sexual nature and arising from the presence of alcohol in the system, which are not known to most persons. So true is this that the writer has thought it well to utter a few words of warning to his women readers concerning these things.

In the first place, there is an exhilarating effect arising from certain kinds of liquor, wines, and other forms of alcoholic drinks, which manifests directly in an excitement of the sexual centers and organism. In many cases a strong sexual excitement, absent at other times, is aroused, and the person is carried away with the force of passion unknown under other circumstances. Added to this the weakened will-power arising from too much drink, and we have an explanation of many cases of "mistakes" of women. It would appear that women are even more susceptible than are men to unusual sexual excitement arising from alcoholic drinks; and that, therefore, they should be especially cautious in the indulgence in such drinks, particularly when in the company of strange men, or men careless in regard to sexual morality and respect for women in their company.

But there is still a deeper reason, based upon the latest discoveries in psychology, why caution in this respect should be observed by women. We allude to the discovery that alcohol first affects the mental and emotional tendencies of more recent racial acquirement, acting so as to paralyze and inhibit the activities thereof, and to thus release the activity of the more primitive emotions and motive activities. Thus, the woman under the influence of alcohol finds that the more recent racial traits, such as sexual control, restraint, sexual morality, conventional observations, etc., are practically temporarily paralyzed in inhibitual—or to use the current slang phrase, are "put out of commission" for the time being; and, at the same time, the old elemental, savage, barbaric, "cave man" instincts, habits, and methods of action, are brought to the surface, and proceed to manifest their activity if opportunity be granted for the same—and the opportunity is usually granted. This being seen to be true, it is seen that the woman so under the influence of liquor is, for the time being, little more than a "cave woman," or barbarian, with all the lax sex morality of the latter, and with all the tendencies to manifest into activity the primitive impulses arising in her nature and demanding expression. Added to this the weakening of will-power always accompanying the alcoholic influence, it is seen that the woman under the influence of strong drink is an easy prey to designing men, and a willing victim to her own lower passions.

An authority of sex subjects says: "That Bacchus, the god of wine, is the strongest ally of Venus, the goddess of love, using the term Love in its physical sense, as the French use the word 'amour,' has been well known to the ancient Greeks and Romans, as it is well known today to every saloon-keeper and every keeper of a disreputable house. And all measures to combat venereal diseases and to prevent girls from making a false step will only be partially successful if we do not at the same time carry on a strong educational campaign against alcoholic indulgence. * * * Of what use are warnings to a girl, when under the influence of a heavy dinner and a bottle of champagne, to which she is unaccustomed, her passion is aroused to a degree she has never experienced before, her will is paralyzed and she yields, though deep down in her consciousness something tells her she shouldn't? She yields, becomes pregnant, and is in the deepest agony for several months, and has a wound which will probably never heal for the rest of her life. Of what use have all the lectures, books, and maternal injunctions been to her? * * * I believe that the sex instinct can be stimulated artificially beyond the natural needs, and among the artificial stimulants of the sex instinct alcohol occupies the first place. And bear in mind that alcohol produces even a stronger effect upon women, in exciting the sexual passion, than it does on men. Women are more easily upset by stimulants and narcotics, and that is the reason why it is more dangerous for women to drink than it is for men. It is impossible to give statistics and exact or even approximate figures. But there is no question in my mind, in the mind of any careful investigator, that if alcoholic beverages could be eliminated, the number of cases of venereal infection would be diminished by about one-half. And what is true of venereal disease is also true of the seduction of young girls. Alcohol is the most efficient weapon that either the refined Don Juan or the vulgar pimp has in his possession."

Our advice to the woman who is asked to drink liquor when in the company of a man outside of her immediate family circle is emphatically this: DON'T DO IT!

The Menstrual Period. As strange as it may appear to those women who have had the advantage of intelligent maternal advice, it is a fact known to all physicians that many mothers permit their young daughters to enter into the stage of puberty, with the accompanying menstrual flow, without having first instructed the daughter as to the meaning and character of this phenomenon of her nature, and without having given her advice concerning the proper care of herself during this period.

Physicians constantly experience cases in which the young girl to whom the first menstrual flow having come, without previous knowledge on her part, has supposed it to be the result of a wound, or of a diseased condition, and has attempted to stop the flow by the application of cold water. Even where a partial knowledge has been attained by the girl, she is found to lack the knowledge of the proper hygienic care of herself during the period. The mothers in such cases are criminally negligent, and have alluded a false modesty or prudery to interfere with a natural and necessary maternal duty.

The approach of the first menstruation is often accompanied by unusual physical, mental and emotional changes in the young girl. Her nervous system is affected, and she is apt to become irritable or morbid, or even somewhat "flighty." Her appetite may become irregular, and there is often present a craving for indigestible food. A physical languor is often experienced, and there may be pains in the back and legs, chilliness and headaches, and a general upsetting of the usual physical condition, accompanied by a manifestation of peevishness and irritability. These unpleasant symptoms usually disappear when the periodical menstrual flow is permanently established. In fact, they are frequently superseded by the awakened energy and heightened spirits of healthy, normal adolescence.

The time of the beginning of the menstrual period varies according to climate, race, condition of health, and temperament. In the tropical countries, menstruation begins from the tenth to the fourteenth year; in temperate countries, from the thirteenth to the sixteenth; in cold countries, from the fifteenth to the twentieth year. The Italian, Hebrew, Spanish, or French girl is apt to menstruate earlier than the English, German, or Swedish girl. The Negro girl menstruates early, as a rule. The full-blooded girl usually menstruates earlier than the anemic one.

Normally, menstruation should proceed naturally and without pain or suffering. When pain or suffering is experienced in connection with menstruation, it is simply because of some lack of health in the general system; and when such general health is restored, the trouble ceases. Painful menstruation is called "dysmenorrhea," and arises from several causes, principal among which are the following: Errors in diet, errors in dress, undue exposure, constipation, lack of proper exercise, or to a contracted or congested condition of the Uterus or the Fallopian Tubes. The pain, however, cannot be considered as a feature of normal menstruation, for the latter is no more painful than a normal movement of the bowels—the painful condition results from abnormal conditions, the removal of these conditions resulting in the cure of the complaint.

Dysmenorrhea should be treated by the discarding of all unhygienic clothing, tight shoes, etc., and their replacement by rational clothing; the dietary should be carefully scanned, and improper articles replaced by nourishing elements of food—discard the pastries, pickles, confections, and stimulants, and substitute sensible articles of diet; if constipation is present, remove it by eating articles of food which promote free movements of the bowels, and drink more water each day; take a proper amount of exercise—housework is as good a form of exercise as any; many authorities advocate the free drinking of water prior to and during the menstrual period—some going so far as to say that **where there is painful menstruation there is always a lack of a proper amount of water taken into the system**. In some cases Dysmenorrhea is due to disorders of the general nervous system, and treatment therefore should be sought at the hands of a capable physician.

Amenorrhea, another disorder arising in connection with the menstrual process, consists of the retention or suppression of the menses, or of "scanty" menses, or occasional "skipping" of the periods. This condition is apt to be manifest in cases of extreme obesity or "fatness;" the nervous system being burdened with superfluous flesh, its menstrual rhythm is often affected. Suppression of the menses also sometimes results from exposure and disturbing mental emotions. The most approved treatment is that of remedying the abnormal general physical condition, proper diet, and the use of hot drinks, hot sitz baths, and hot enemas about the time of the beginning of the normal period.

Menorrhagia, another menstrual-period disorder, consists of very profuse flowing—it is, in fact, a mild form of hemorrhage. It usually arises from general debility, shocks, too violent exercise or labor, and also in many cases from undue and too frequent sexual intercourse. Sometimes the excessive flow occurs during the regular menstrual period, while in other cases it may manifest itself out of season—sometimes as often as two or three times a month. The duration of the normal period of menstrual flow, however, varies greatly among different women; the normal period may be said to last from two to six days, so what might be an excessive flow for one woman would be only normal for another—temperament plays a large part in determining the quantity of the menses.

Some of the accompanying symptoms of Menorrhagia, or profuse flow, are lassitude, shortness of breath, faintness, dizziness, headache, irritability and nervousness, and often also leucorrhea between periods. The general treatment consists in measures calculated to bring the general health of the woman back to the normal. The building up of the general system, by means of nourishing food, proper exercise, etc., will almost always result in curing this disorder.

A well-known authority has well said: "The hygiene of menstruation can be expressed in two words: **Cleanliness and Rest**."

So far as Rest is concerned, the woman need not be urged to take it at this period—that is, if she is able to do so. Care should be taken not to exercise unduly at this time, and under the head of exercise may be included dancing, horseback riding, and automobiling, as well as the more common forms of athletic work.

It would seem that common sense and the general desire for cleanliness and daintiness would cause all women to observe the plain hygienic laws of Cleanliness at the time of the menstrual period. And, indeed, it is probable that such would be the case were it not for the fact that some ancient superstitions still exert their power over the mind of many women, in regard to the use of water during the menstrual period. While it is true that cold baths, or cold-water bathing, are not advisable for the average woman during the menstrual period (although some especially robust women bathe and swim as usual during this period), this prohibition does not apply to the use of **warm** water during the period. Lukewarm baths are permissible at this time; and the woman should wash the external genital parts with warm water, with soap if desired, every morning and evening of the period. A vaginal douche of lukewarm water is an excellent adjunct to the bathing of the parts.

It is astonishing to meet with the superstitious prejudice existing in the minds of some women concerning the use of the vaginal douche; these good creatures seem to think that it is either unnatural and unhealthy, or else is something "not respectable," and fit only for the use of immoral women.

These women should get in touch with modern hygienic methods, and learn to use the douche at least during their menstrual periods. At this time, if the plain rules of cleanliness are not observed, there often occurs a decomposition of the blood which has gathered in or about the genitals, and an offensive odor is manifested. Some women, while feeling distressed about this odor, are afraid to use lukewarm water in washing themselves, owing to some old unexplored superstition handed down from the great-grandmother's time.

The napkins should be changed at least every morning and evening. Unclean napkins may lead to infection, and it is probable that many cases of leucorrhea have their origin in lack of cleanliness concerning the napkins, cloths, or rags, used during menstruation. It may seem almost incredible to the average woman reader, but physicians know of cases (usually among the poorer and more ignorant foreign classes) in which the girl is instructed by her mother, grandmother, or aunts, that she must wear the original cloth or rag during the entire period, as she will "catch cold" by a change to a clean, fresh cloth while the flow continued. Imagine the result of such a practice! This last is an extreme instance, of course, but it will serve to show the absurd and harmful notions prevalent concerning this important natural function, and its incidents.

Leucorrhea. A very common disorder among women is that known as Leucorrhea, or "the whites." It consists of a discharge from the Vagina, or the Uterus through the Vagina. It is, in fact, of a catarrhal nature, and results from an over-secretion of the mucus fluids which, in proper quantity, keep the mucus membrane of the said organs in good condition. The discharge manifests in various shades and degrees of consistency. From the character of the discharge, physicians are able to determine whether it comes from the Vagina or the Uterus. The discharge from the Vagina usually is a light creamy fluid; that from the neck of the Uterus is a sticky, thick fluid flowing rather freely; that from the lining of the Uterus is alkaline, and generally precedes and follows menstruation; and that accompanying ulceration of the womb is semi-purulent and offensive in odor.

Leucorrhea has many causes, among which may be mentioned the following: getting chilled feet or body, particularly during the menstrual period; over exertion and overwork standing on one's feet; chills following dancing in overheated rooms; excessive worry or emotional strain, etc. It is a quite common complaint, and some assert that fully twenty-five per cent (perhaps more) of all women suffer from it to at least some extent.

The general treatment of Leucorrhea consists of the building up of the entire system by the proper hygienic methods. Constipation should be removed, and the system is built up by the proper articles of food, exercise, etc. The use of the proper douches are also advised by the best practitioners. Physicians also treat inflamed areas by local treatments consisting of painting the Vagina or neck of the Uterus with certain medicinal solutions. Certain suppositories and douches are also employed in some cases. It is always better to consult a good physician in these cases, particularly where the trouble is aggravated or of long standing.

A popular writer on the subject gives the following prescription for a vaginal injection: White Fluid Hydrastics, 2 ounces; Borax, 1/2 ounce; Distilled Witch Hazel Extract, 1 pint. Use of this preparation **one ounce, diluted in a pint of lukewarm water**, as a vaginal injection, taken twice each day.

A well-known authority gives the following advice concerning treatment of Leucorrhea: "One of the simplest things is an alum tampon. You take a piece of absorbent cotton, about the size of a fist, spread it out, put about a tablespoonful of powdered alum on it, fold it up, tie a string around the center, insert it in the vagina as far as it will go, and leave it in twenty-four hours. Then pull it gently by the string and syringe yourself with a quart or two of warm water. Such a tampon may be inserted every other day or every third day, and I have known where this simple treatment alone produced a cure. In some cases, however, douches work better, and the two best things for douching are: tincture of iodine and lactic acid. Buy, say, four ounces of tincture of iodine, and use two teaspoonsful in two quarts of hot water in a douche bag. This injection should be used twice a day, morning and night. Of the lactic acid you buy, say, a pint, and use two tablespoonsful to two quarts of water. The lactic acid has the advantage over the tincture of iodine that it is colorless, while the iodine is dark and stains whatever it comes in contact with. Sometimes I order the use of the tincture of iodine and the lactic acid alternately: for one douche the tincture of iodine, for the next the lactic acid, and so on. When the condition improves, it is sufficient to use one teaspoonful of the tincture of iodine and one tablespoonful of the lactic acid to two quarts of water. These injections are quite efficient and have the advantage of being perfectly harmless. One point about the injections: they should be taken not in the standing or squatting position (in which position the fluid comes right out), but while laying down, over a douche pan. The douche bag should be only about a foot above the bed, so that the irrigating fluid may come out slowly; the patient, after each injection taken in the daytime, should remain at least half an hour in bed (in the nighttime she stays all night in bed.) This gives the injection a better chance to come in contact with all the parts of the vagina, and a portion of it comes in contact with the cervix, where it exerts a healing effect. Avoid the use of patent medicines."

Uterine Displacement. The woman suffering from Uterine Displacement should, of course, consult a competent physician and be governed by his advice. The following suggestions, however, will be found to be of service in many cases:

In the case of **Prolapsus,** or falling of the womb, many women have found great relief, and in many cases permanent improvement, by taking occasional rests in bed for an hour or so, with the feet and lower part of the legs raised at least eight inches above the level of the head. In this plan, the Uterus is replaced by gravitation. Some authorities advise practicing waist-breathing while lying in this position, thus exercising the abdominal muscles. Dr. Taylor says: "Increase the pump-like action of the chest, and it will be found that the displaced viscera will return to their normal position." Some have also found relief from the use of alum-water vaginal injections once or twice each day. The alum-water is prepared by dissolving one heaping teaspoonful of powdered alum in a pint of lukewarm water. This last treatment often strengthens the vaginal muscles whose yielding has at least partially been the cause of the falling womb.

In cases of **Retroversion**, in which the Uterus is turned or bent backward, the "knee and chest" position will often aid in causing the organ to regain its normal position. In this position the woman kneels, and rests her chest upon the bed, thus causing the hips to be elevated.

In cases of **Antroversion**, in which the Uterus is turned or bent forward, relief is often obtained by the woman resting upon the back, using a pillow to elevate her hips.

Intercourse During Menstruation. It would seem that the natural esthetic repulsion to the exercise of the marital relations during the menstrual period should be sufficient to deter men and women from indulgence at this time; but many seem to have overcome this instinctive repulsion, and to these a stronger reason must be given—and the reason is at hand. The reasons in question are as follows: first, that congestion of the Uterus and Ovaries sometimes results from this unnatural practice; second, that the man may possibly contract an inflammation of the urethra by infection from the degenerated membrane, tissue, blood, etc., of the menstrual flow; and third, that such practices may result in the aggravation of discharges from the woman, such as leucorrhea, etc.

Intercourse During Pregnancy. The best authorities advise total abstinence from sexual intercourse during the period of pregnancy; but in view of the fact that such abstinence is very difficult for most men, and that few will persist in it, it is thought well to point out the fact that at least an extreme moderation is desirable in such cases. A leading authority says on this point: "During the first four months of pregnancy, no change need be made in the usual sex relations; their intensity should be moderated, their frequency need not. During the fifth, sixth, and seventh months, intercourse should be indulged in at rarer intervals—once in two or three weeks—the act should be performed without any violence or intensity. During the eighth and ninth months relations had best be given up altogether. And this abstinence should last until about six weeks after the birth of the child. During this period the uterus undergoes what we call involution; that is, it goes back to the size and shape it had before pregnancy, and it is best not to disturb this process by sexual excitement, which causes engorgement and congestion."

Sterility in Women. Sterility, or barrenness, i. e., the inability to bear children, is frequently met with among married people. It is usually blamed upon the woman, whereas in at least one-half of the cases the fault is with the man.

The causes of sterility in women are usually one or more of the following: Inflammation of the Fallopian Tubes, which may have been caused by gonorrhea or ordinary inflammation—in some rare cases childbirth has been known to set up an inflammation in this region, which has prevented the woman from future childbearing—the inflammation causes the tubes to clog up or become closed, so that no more ova can pass through them from the ovaries to the womb; in some cases, also, severe cases of leucorrhea have caused sterility, as the discharge is sometimes fatal to the life of the spermatozoa and destroys them; in other cases misplacement of the womb causes sterility; also severe inflammation of the neck or mouth of the womb operates in the same way, in some cases. In cases of sterility, the woman should have an examination made by a competent physician, and it often will be found that the cure of the disorders above noted will work a cure of the sterility.

But, in all cases of sterility, it will be found that the husband should be examined as well as the wife—in fact, many authorities insist that the husband should be examined first. Venereal diseases frequently produce sterility in the man, although he is loath to admit this and is apt to place the blame entirely upon the woman.

Miscarriage and Abortions. The terms "miscarriage," and "abortion," respectively, mean the expulsion of the fetus from the womb before its natural time of delivery. In common usage, the term "miscarriage" is usually employed to indicate instances in which the premature delivery has occurred without any voluntary act on the part of the woman, or other persons acting with her permission; the term "abortion" being reserved for instances in which the miscarriage has been voluntarily produced.

When the fetus dies within the womb of the mother, it is usually expelled spontaneously within a few days or even a few hours. Some women suffer from certain weakness which result in habitual miscarriage; such women seem unable to carry the child for the full natural term, and lose it at some time during the period of gestation. Like results often arise from certain diseases, principal among which is syphilis. In some cases the physician produces what is known as "therapeutic abortion," for the purpose of saving the life of the woman—this is sanctioned by medical custom and by law. Other forms of abortion, performed for the purpose of preventing the progress of the gestation, and designed for the destruction of the embryo or fetus, are known as "criminal abortion," and are punishable by several legal penalties.

Abortions are frequently followed by severe illness, invalidism, or even death for the woman. Many women have had their entire lives ruined by this evil practice. It is one of the curses of modern civilization, and one which must be removed by means of rational instruction and education along the lines of sexual science if the race is to be prevented from deterioration. The subject will be further considered in the subsequent lessons in this book.

The best advice to those who have contemplated the performance of abortion is simply this: Don't; **Don't**; **DON'T!**

LESSON VI
THE SCIENCE OF EUGENICS

No one who keeps in even only fair touch with the affairs of the world of today can have failed to notice the frequent mention of the term "Eugenics" in the newspapers, magazine, and books of the hour. And yet, many persons seem to be in doubt as to the meaning and use of the term; some thinking that it refers to some new "ism" or "ology," or perhaps to some new and strange doctrine concerning the relations of the sexes. In view of this fact, the writer has thought it well to give the readers of this book a brief, though somewhat comprehensive, view of the general subject of Eugenics.

Eugenics, sometimes known as the Science of Parenthood, has well been styled "the New Science," for it has forced itself into public notice within the past ten or fifteen years, whereas before that time it was practically unknown to the general public. At the present time some of the world's greatest thinkers have spoken or written on the subject, and many regard it as one of the most vital branches of human research, endeavor, and study, for the future of the race is involved in the solution of its problems. In its general phase of race-betterment, Eugenics is receiving the attention of statesmen, sociologists and patriots; in its particular phases, the earnest attention, interest and study of men and women who wish offspring of the best quality obtainable.

The spirit of Eugenics may be expressed in the words of Dr. G. Stanley Hall, president of Clark University, who has said: "Our duty of all duties is to transmit the sacred torch of life undiminished, and, if possible, a little brightened, to our children. This is the chief end of men and women. All posterity slumbers in our bodies, as we did in our ancestors. The basis of the new biological ethics of today, and of the future, is that everything is right that makes for the welfare of the yet unborn, and all is wrong that injures them, and to do so is the unpardonable sin—the only one nature knows."

That phase of Eugenics which has brought the new science more prominently before the public mind, and which has enrolled on its roster the names of some of the world's most eminent scientists, sociologists, and writers—the phase of race-betterment from the standpoint of sociology—has led many to believe that Eugenics is confined to that phase, and is but a movement toward "the successful breeding of the human race" on a universal scale. To many, such a movement while deemed commendable and desirable nevertheless lacks the appeal of the heart and affections—it seems to be of the head alone. But when such persons are brought to their realization that Eugenics is also a movement to promote the bearing of children—to enable each mated couple to bring forth perfect offspring—then the heart is enlisted as a co-worker with the head.

The sociological phase of Eugenics—the phase of Race Culture in general—is being vigorously advanced by societies and organizations in various parts of the world, the parent organization being the Eugenics Education Society, of London, England. Dr. C. W. Saleeby, one of those prominent in the work of the said Society, has the following to say concerning the work of that organization:

"The Eugenics Education Society exists to uphold the ideal of Parenthood as the highest and most responsible of human powers; to proclaim that the racial instinct is therefore supremely sacred, and its exercise through marriage, for the service of the future, the loftiest of all privileges. It stands for a transfigured sentiment of parenthood which regards with solicitude not child and grandchild only, but the generations to come hereafter—fathers of the future creating and providing for the remote children. That which too many schools of thought and practice have derided or defiled, it seeks to elevate and ennoble. Parenthood on the part of the diseased, the insane, the alcoholic—where these conditions promise to be transmitted—must be denounced as a crime against the future. In these directions the Society stands for active legislation, and for the formation of that public opinion which legislation, if it is to be effective, must express. Parenthood on the part of the worthy must be buttressed, guided, and extolled. The Society stands for the education of the young regarding the responsibility and holiness of the racial function of parenthood."

The Eugenists hold that in the near future our children, looking back upon the present and the past state of indifference and neglect concerning the important subject of bearing and rearing of children, will experience the same horror that we now feel when we look back upon the indifference to the horrors of human slavery, imprisonment for debt, cruelty toward prisoners, treatment of the insane, executions for trivial offences, etc., on the part of our ancestors. Our descendants will deem it almost inconceivable that we, their ancestors, could have been so blind and criminally negligent.

But, as leading Eugenists have pointed out, the new science does not confine its attention to the subject of preventive measures, important as they are—it also directs its attention to the constructive phase of the subject, i. e., the production of better children. While Eugenics strives to prevent the unfit from flooding the race with unfit progeny, it at the same time strives to educate the race so that the fit may bear and rear better offsprings. It is not sufficient merely to eliminate the unfit—we must also improve, and still further render fit, the fit members of the race. The fit must not be allowed to remain merely the fit—we must evolve a fitter—and ever move onward toward the realization of the ideal of the fittest. We must not only strive to eliminate the beast in the race of men—we must also aid the race to unfold in the direction of the super-man.

The Eugenists know that much of the talk concerning Race Suicide is not only futile and uncalled for, but is also in a sense misleading and actually dangerous. The real danger of Race Suicide comes not from the decreasing birth-rate, but from the excessive, ignorant, and unscientific bearing and rearing of children by unfit parents. It is not so much a matter of **how many** children are born, as of **how** they are born, what kind of children they are, and how they are reared physically, mentally and morally, and how many survive. It is not so much that the lower death-rate be avoided, says the Eugenist, as it is that the higher death-rate be overcome. The intelligent stockbreeder grasps this scientific law of the Eugenists when he endeavors to produce the best young, and then to take care of them that they survive and reach a healthy maturity. To the Eugenist, it is not so much a question of "more," but of "better"—not so much a question of quantity as of quality —not so much a question of production, but of conservation and preservation.

Dr. Saleeby refers to the death-rate of London, which is but 16 to the 1000, as compared to that of Bombay, which is 79 to the 1000. He adds: "It is asserted that in many large Indian cities the infant mortality approaches one-half of all the children born. What it amounts to in such cities as Canton and Pekin we can only surmise with horror. * * * * Unless it be supposed by bishops and others, then, that a peculiar value attaches to the production of a baby shortly to be buried, the suggestion evidently is the same as that to which every humanitarian and social and patriotic impulse guides us, namely, the reduction of the death-rate, and especially of infant mortality. * * * * Hence the Eugenists and the Episcopal Bench may join hands so far as the reduction of the death-rate is concerned, and the only persons with whom a practical quarrel remains are those who applaud the mother who boasts that she has buried twelve."

The Eugenists urge that if the principles applied to plant-life by that master of his science, Luther Burbank, were applied to the production and rearing of young human life, in a few generations we should have a race so far advanced beyond the present average as to be almost god-like by comparison. But this means a far different thing from the ideal of merely "more children"—it requires the manifestation of the ideal of "better children," well born, carefully reared, well nourished, and scientifically educated. And this rearing, nourishing, and education must not be confined to the physical part of the child's nature—it must proceed along the three-fold line of physical, mental, and moral culture.

The Eugenists have been actively concerned with the question of the prevention of the transmission of undesirable qualities to offspring. They have held that while crime is more frequently rather the result of evil environment than of criminal heredity, nevertheless there is a large class of children who are "born criminals"—that is, born with such a decided tendency toward criminal acts that the slightest influence of environment may, and often does, serve to kindle into a blaze the undesirable and criminal characteristics.

Dr. Saleeby says of this: "In the face of the work of Lombroso and his school, exaggerated though some of their conclusions may be, we cannot dispute the existence of born criminals and the criminal type. There are undoubtedly many such persons in modern society. There is an abundance of crime which no education, practiced or imaginable, would eliminate. Present day psychology and medicine and, for the matter of that, ordinary common-sense, can readily distinguish cases at both extremes—the mattoid or semi-insane criminal at one end, and the decent citizen who yields to exceptional temptation at the other end."

The Eugenists quote as an instance of the above contention the celebrated case of Max Jukes, a notorious criminal and drunkard, who as the records show us was the ancestor of a foul brood of descendants which cost the State of New York over a million dollars in seventy-five years. Among these descendants were 200 thieves and murderers; 285 subject to idiocy, blindness or deafness; 90 prostitutes; and 300 children born prematurely. It is possible that a portion of this evil result was caused not alone by bad heredity but, at least in part, by the suggestion of the environment, and the influence of example of the parents; but even so, the primal cause was that Max Jukes, the notoriously unfit ancestor, was allowed to propagate this evil brood, destined to be born and reared under the most adverse conditions and environment.

The Eugenists also place great importance upon the prevention of insane persons becoming parents. To those who consider that this is but an exceptional and rare occurrence, the Eugenists reply that a large percentage of insane patients in asylums have a family history showing insanity in one or both parents; that reports show that there are thousands of feeble-minded women in every large city allowed to (yes, often actually compelled to) bear children to their husbands or male companions.

Ribot says: "Every work on insanity is a plea for heredity." Maudsley says: "More than one-fourth and less than one-half of all insanity is heredity." Riddell says: "Of the great causes of insanity, alcoholism is perhaps the greatest, while morbid heredity ranks next. Insanity is largely the result of degeneracy. Most persons who become mentally deranged are the offspring of neurotic, drunken, insane or feeble-minded parents." While it by no means follows that one must manifest traits of insanity or mental disturbance simply because one of his parents suffered from a like trouble —and we believe that many a one has frightened himself into those conditions by pure auto-suggestion inspired by a one-sided belief in heredity—still it is unquestionably true that a fair mind must concede that wisdom and a proper sense of right and justice would require that parents of unsound mental tendencies should not be permitted to bring into the world children who might inherit a tendency toward a like, or worse, condition.

The Eugenists also have called the attention of the thinking public to the danger of deaf-and-dumb persons transmitting their condition to their offspring. Of this Dr. Saleeby says: "The condition known as deaf-mutism is congenital or due to innate defect in about one-half of all the cases in Great Britain." Dr. Love says: "In every institution, examples may be found of deaf-mute children who have had one or two deaf parents or grandparents, and of two or more deaf-mute children belonging to one family." A case is noted in England where a deaf-and-dumb man having been killed by an accident, his relatives could not identify the body, as the wife and sister were blind, deaf-and-dumb, and the four children were deaf-and-dumb. The man and his wife were both deaf-and-dumb when they were married, the wife being also blind.

Perhaps no subject has aroused the active Eugenists to a greater pitch of indignation than the ascertained results of the effect upon offspring of parents addicted to the over-indulgence in alcohol. It is known by the records that a large number of cases of feeble-mindedness and actual insanity are due to inebriety of parents, and often of grandparents, or ancestors for several generations. Epilepsy, idiocy, and criminality are also traceable in many cases to drunkenness of parents. Dr. Saleeby, moved by indignation by the ascertained results of the investigations of the Eugenists, has said: "Parenthood must be forbidden to the dipsomaniac, the chronic inebriate, or the drunkard, whether male or female."

Professor Grenier, writing on the subject of alcoholic degeneration, has said: "Alcohol is one of the most active agents in the degeneracy of the race. The indelible effects produced by heredity are not to be remedied. Alcoholic descendants are often inferior beings, a notable proportion coming under the categories of idiots, imbeciles, and the debilitated. The morbid influence of parents is maximum when conception has taken place at the time of drunkenness of one or both parties. Those with hereditary alcoholism show a tendency to excess; half of them become alcoholics; a large number of cases of neurosis have their principal cause in alcoholic antecedents. The larger portion of the sons of alcoholics have convulsions in early infancy. Epilepsy is almost characteristic of the alcoholism of parents, when it is not an index of a nervous disposition of the whole family. The alcoholic delirium is more frequent in the descendants of alcoholics than in their parents, which indicates their intellectual degeneration."

What has been said of alcoholism of course applies to the use of narcotics and other drugs. Galton cites a case in which "a man who had had two healthy children acquired the cocaine habit, and while suffering from the symptoms of chronic poisoning engendered two idiots." And yet had anyone publicly instructed the wife of this man regarding the use of contraceptives, such person would have been liable to imprisonment!

Another subject engaging the active attention of the Eugenists, and which is discussed to considerable extent in the privacy of their meetings, but which must be voiced only very carefully in the public prints owing to the "murderous silence" which society prefers to maintain on the subject, is of the influence of venereal diseases as racial poisons transmissible to offspring. Dr. Saleeby has well said: "No other disease can rival syphilis in its hideous influence upon parenthood and the future. But it is no crime for a man to marry, infect his innocent bride and their children; no crime against the laws of our lawgivers, but a heinous outrage against nature's decrees. When at last our laws are based on nature's laws, criminal marriages of this kind may be put an end to."

The above stated facts are not pleasant reading for most persons, and many pass over them hurriedly, thereby hoping to escape the mental discomfort which the hearing and learning of unpleasant truths so often produce. But the subject will not down—it is forcing itself to the attention of the thinking members of society today in a manner which will admit of no escape. These facts must be faced, and steps must be taken by society to protect the race from degeneration and actual Race Suicide. And the Science of Eugenics is pointing the way.

Dr. Saleeby says of this phase of Eugenics: "Negative Eugenics will seek to define the diseases and defects which are really hereditary; to name those the transmission of which is already known to occur, and to raise the average of the race by interfering as far as may be with the parenthood of persons suffering from these transmissible disorders. Only thus can certain of the gravest evils of society, as, for instance, feeble-mindedness, insanity, and crime due to inherited degeneracy, be suppressed; and if Race-Culture were absolutely incapable of effecting anything whatever in the way of increasing the fertility of the worthiest classes and individuals, its services in the negative direction here briefly outlined would be of incalculable value. To this policy we shall most certainly come; but here, as in other cases, I trust far more to the influence of an educated public opinion than in legislation; though there are certain forms of transmissible disease, interfering in no way with the responsibility of the individual, the transmission of which should be visited with the utmost rigor of the law, and regarded as utterly criminal, no less than sheer murder."

But the Science of Eugenics is concerned not only with telling society what "not to do"—it is equally concerned with telling it "what to do." It has its Positive as well as its Negative side. After pointing out the evils of procreation on the part of the unfit, it then proceeds to tell the fit how to best serve the interests of the unborn. Eugenics is not satisfied with merely plucking out the foul weeds which have encumbered the fair garden of life —it seeks also to furnish to the real flowers better soil, and improved conditions, and to give them the benefit of the best selection, breeding and conditions, that they may evolve and improve into still more glorious products of nature's power.

The Eugenists earnestly advocate laws and public opinion tending to protect mothers and expectant mothers. They recognize the supremacy of motherhood, and aim to encourage and protect it. They decry the common indifference toward this function which is all important in the preservation and evolution of the race, and which neglect is well expressed in the complaint of Bouchacourt, who said: "The dregs of the human species—the blind, the deaf-mute, the degenerate, the imbecile, the epileptic—are better protected than are pregnant women."

The Eugenists believe in educating women for motherhood, and in protecting them from conditions which interfere with that important function of their life. They are not fully agreed upon the methods to be pursued in cases of expectant mothers whose lack of proper support prevents them from obtaining the proper nourishment, etc., but in a general way it may be said that they agree in holding that the expectant mother should be looked upon as the honored ward of the State, and should be properly provided for from the public funds.

The Eugenists also believe in educating the father, or prospective father. They hold that every man should be made acquainted with the duties and responsibilities of fatherhood, and should so conduct and order his life that the production and rearing of a family should result as a consummation of a long cherished ideal. The man should be taught to prepare himself, physically, mentally, and morally, for his coming responsibility to the race. He should also be taught to respect and regard motherhood, and to make it his business to secure and preserve the best possible conditions for the mother of his own children, and the mothers of other men's children, not as an act of mere sentiment, but as a public duty, a patriotic service, a racial obligation.

The Eugenists believe in teaching young men and young women on the subject of sexual physiology and psychology. They hold that the race is now criminally negligent in such matters, and that young men and women, by the thousands, enter into the state of marriage and parenthood with no knowledge regarding the sacred functions which they are to bring into activity. They believe that the first requisite of scientific parenthood is and must be a sane knowledge of the physiology of sex, and the psychology of sex. There must be sane education concerning the sexual organism, its laws, its functions, its normal and healthy condition, its anatomy, physiology and hygiene.

The average physician of several years' experience can tell tales of almost incredible ignorance on the part of persons who have recently entered into the relationship of marriage. In some cases the ignorance is more than a mere absence of knowledge, for it consists of an array of false-knowledge, untruthful ideas, of often serious importance. It is sad enough to think how the ignorance and false-knowledge may work results hurtful to the young couple themselves, but it is even sadder to realize that these same ignorant or wrongly-informed young persons must gain their real knowledge through sad experience which is to be paid for not only by themselves but also by their children. It is a hard saying, but true that "the knowledge of the majority of young parents is gained by experience paid for by their unborn children."

The Eugenists look forward to the coming of the day when it will be regarded as reprehensible to allow young persons to enter into the relationship of marriage without a sane, practical knowledge of their own reproductive organism and functions, and of their physiological duties to themselves, their companions in marriage, and to their children born or to be born. We may, in due time, see a practical realization of the ideal set forth by Dr. Newell Dwight Hillis, who said: "The State that makes a man study two years before a license as druggist is given; that makes a young lawyer or doctor study three years before being permitted to practice, ought to ask the young man or young woman to pass an equally rigid examination before license is given to found an American home, and set up an American family."

This idea of the scientific preparation for parenthood is a new one for many, but the coming generations will recognize its importance to the individual and to the race. Many who recognize the influence of pre-natal culture in so far as is concerned the physical, mental, and moral condition of the mother during pregnancy, have failed to perceive that an equally important influence is exerted by the physical, mental and moral condition of **both parents** before the conception of the child. These conditions are reflected, often very markedly, in the child, and an avoidance of consideration in this respect is often almost criminal negligence.

Eugenists deplore the haphazard way in which children are so often conceived. More care is often bestowed upon the conditions precedent to the conception of the domestic animals than is given by their owners to the conditions preceding the conception of their own offspring. Too often, while in the case of the domestic animals the utmost care is exercised regarding the arrangement for the breeding of valuable stock, the human offspring are mere "accidents," conceived without intention, forethought, or preparation; and too often is such conception undesired, regretted and unwelcome.

This state of affairs is utterly unworthy of civilized man with the knowledge of science at his command, and the intellect and will with which to carry out the plain dictates of reason and duty. Nature does her part unhindered in the case of the lower animals, and man should use her principles as a foundation upon which to build a structure which reason and intelligence should supply the materials. Instead of this, man too often discards Nature's plain rules entirely, and also refuses to use his reason, and, instead, allows himself to be ruled by selfish inclinations and desires, and ignoble motives.

To those who may ask: "But why should we give all this time, care and trouble to the young of the race—what is their claim upon us that demands so much of us in return for so little on their part?" the answer is plain. We should do this not alone because of the natural feeling of love for our own offspring which is innate in all normal human beings, but we should also do this because we owe a duty to the race in and which we are units—a duty which demands that we supply to the race the best material, and only the best, for its preservation, continuance, and betterment.

The spirit of the age is pointing out the direction indicated by Eugenics and scientific Birth Control. And it is a spirit in which the best mental and spiritual powers of man are called into action. A new consciousness—the "race consciousness"—is awakening within the best of the race, and accompanying it is a new **conscience**—a "race conscience"—is manifesting within us, and is giving the individual a sense of right and wrong toward future generations, just as his earlier-awakened social conscience has opened his eyes to his duties toward his neighbors.

Man is beginning to feel that all men are his brothers, and that the future generations of men are in a sense his children. The new ideal of "Let us build posterity worthily" has begun to supplant the old narrow idea humorously expressed in the famous bull of Sir Boyce Roche, who said, "Why should we do anything for posterity—what has posterity ever done for us?"

As Dr. Saleeby has well said: "If the struggle toward individual perfection be religious, so assuredly is the struggle, less egoistic indeed, toward racial perfection. * * * And they that shall be of us shall build up the old waste places; for we shall raise up the foundations of many generations."

And in all this, also, we find ever present the distinctive note of modern thought, viz., "**Not more children, but better ones; not more births, but less deaths and more survivals; not numerical birth values, but qualitative birth values and numerical survival values.**"

LESSON VII
PRE-NATAL INFLUENCES

The term "Pre-Natal" of course means "before birth," and Pre-Natal Influences are those influences exerted upon the child before its birth into the world. The students of Eugenics are vitally interested in the subject of Pre-Natal Influences, as they recognize that therein is to be found the secret of much which will work along the line of "better offspring," and general race-betterment.

Pre-Natal Influences (as the term is used in the present consideration of the subject) may be considered as manifesting in three phases, as follows:

(1) The influence of the physical, mental, and moral "family characteristics" of the parents, transmitted to the child along the lines of heredity.

(2) The influence of the acquired personal characteristics of the parents (particularly the acquired characteristics which are especially active at and just previous to the time of actual conception), transmitted to the child along the lines of heredity.

(3) The influence of "maternal impressions" (after conception, and during the period of gestation or pregnancy) transmitted to the child physiologically and psychologically.

I shall now ask you to proceed with me to a consideration of the various phases of Pre-Natal Influences coming under the above name three general classes, and the principal factors involved therein.

Heredity in General.

By "heredity" is meant "the tendency which there is in each animal or plant, in all essential characters, to resemble its parents"; or "the hereditary transmission of physical or psychical characteristics of parents to their offspring."

There is a great disagreement among the authorities as to how far the principle of heredity really extends, and the real causes of heredity are in dispute. In the present consideration we shall, of course, pass over the technical phases of the subject, and shall touch only upon the general features and principles involved.

Shute, in his work entitled "Organic Evolution," says: "That an offspring always inherits from its parents many of their characteristics is well known; that it always varies, more or less, from them, is also equally well known. Heredity and variation are twin forces that play upon every creature, holding it rigidly true to the parental type or compelling more or less divergence therefrom, according to the strength of the one or other power; so that every creature is the resultant of the activities of these two great parallel forces. Variation is co-extensive with heredity, and every living creature gives evidence of the existence of variations.

"Mental heredity can be illustrated by studying the genealogies of such persons as Aristotle, Goethe, Darwin, Coleridge, Milton, etc. Probably the Bach family, of Germany, supply one of the best illustrations of the inheritance of intellectual character that we know of. The record of this family begins in 1550, lasting through eight generations to 1800. For about two centuries it gave to the world musicians and singers of high rank. The founder was Weit Bach, a baker of Presburg, who sought recreation from his routine work in song and music. For nearly two hundred years his descendants, who were very numerous in Franconia, Thuringia, and Saxony, retained a musical talent, being all church singers and organists. When the members of the family had become very numerous and widely separated from one another, they decided to meet at a stated place once a year. Often more than a hundred persons—men, women, and children—bearing the name of Bach were thus brought together. This family reunion continued until nearly the middle of the eighteenth century. In this family of musicians, twenty-nine became eminent.

"Inheritance of moral character is well known. Heredity, in its relation to crime and pauperism, has been thoroughly investigated by Mr. Dugdale in his most instructive little work entitled "The Jukes." In this work the descendants of one vicious and neglected girl are traced through a large number of generations. It reveals that a large proportion of the descendants of this woman became licentious, for, in the course of six generations, fifty-two percent of the children were illegitimate. It shows also that there were seven times more paupers among the women than among the average women of the state, and nine times more paupers among the male descendants than among the average men of the state. The inheritance of physical peculiarities is so obvious as to need no illustration. Among the ancients the Romans stereotyped its truth by the use of such expressions as 'the labiones' or thick-lipped; 'the nasones,' or big-nosed; 'the capitones,' or big-headed, and 'the buccones,' or swollen-cheeked, etc. In more recent times we read of the Austrian lip and the Bourbon nose."

But in all considerations of the subject of heredity, one must always remember that the inheritance of physical, mental, and moral characteristics is not alone from the immediate parents, but rather from many ancestors further removed in order and time. Back of each person there is a long line of paternal and maternal ancestors, extending back to the beginning of the race. And in that line there are influences for good and evil, awaiting favorable environment for awakening into new life unless restrained by the will of the individual.

As Shute says: "There will come a time when the fertilized ovum will have a highly complex nucleus composed of many different ancestral groups of hereditary units. One often hears the expression that a child is a chip of the old block; but this is only a very partial truth, for the child is pre-eminently a composite chip of many old blocks." And Luther Burbank has well said: "Heredity means much; but what is heredity? Not some hideous ancestral spectre, forever crossing the path of a human being. Heredity is simply the sum of all the environments of all past generations on the responsive ever-moving life-forces."

Transmission of Acquired Characteristics.

One of the great disputes of biology is that concerning the question of whether or not parents may transmit to their offspring their personal "acquired characteristics" as well as those inherited from their line of ancestors. One side of the controversy points to the observed cases of children and grandchildren resembling each other, physically, mentally, and morally, in acquired characteristics; but the other side explains these facts as due to environment rather than to heredity.

The best authorities seem to favor a middle-view, holding that acquired characteristics may be and are transmitted as "tendencies" in the offspring. Thus as each succeeding generation manifests the acquired tendency, it adds a cumulative force to the family heredity. At the same time they hold that "environment" is needed to "draw out" the inherited "tendency." For instance, a child born with evil tendencies, and placed in an evil environment, will most likely manifest evil conduct. The same child, if placed in a good environment, will not have the evil tendencies "drawn out" by the environment, and will probably not manifest evil conduct. The same rule applies to the child drawn with good "tendencies." In short, it is held that heredity and environment tend to balance each other—the "something within" is called out (or not called out) by the "something without." The life of the individual is held to be a continuous action and reaction between heredity and environment, and both of these elements must be taken into consideration when we think of the subject.

Shute says: "As influencing a man's life and character, which is the strongest factor, heredity or environment?" In our opinion, as the result of long study and reading, where we have an average man of a sound mind in a sound body, there environment will be the strongest factor whether for good or evil—that is, in men in general, who have no organic defect, such as insanity or idiocy, and allied affections, the stronger force is environment; but in those having such defect, heredity is the controlling power, and we may add, the destroying power.

The Eugenic Rule Regarding Heredity.

It is one of the cardinal principles of Eugenics that those with a bad family history should not become parents. By this it is not meant that the manifestation of undesirable tendencies, physical, mental, and moral, on the part of certain individuals of a family necessarily constitutes a "bad family history." On the contrary, many of the best families have, from time to time, individuals who manifest undesirable tendencies, and who are in general out of harmony with the general family standard. It is an old axiom that "there is a black sheep in every flock"; and the flock must be measured by its general standard, and not by its exceptional black sheep.

A "bad family history" is one in which the family has clearly manifested certain undesirable physical, mental, and moral traits in a marked degree, and in a sufficient number of instances to establish a standard. Some families have a "bad family history" for inebriety; others for epilepsy; others for licentiousness; others for dishonesty—the history extending over several generations, and including a marked number of individuals in each generation. Individuals of such a family should refrain from bearing children; and if children be born to such the greatest care should be exercised by the parents in the matter of surrounding the child with the environment least calculated to "draw out" the undesirable characteristic. The child has a right to be well born, and to be protected from being brought into the world subjected to the handicap of a "bad family history." If individuals cannot endow their children with a good family history, they should refrain from bearing children—such is the Eugenic advice on the subject.

The same rule applies to the question of "acquired characteristics" of the parents—especially those acquired characteristics which are especially active at or just before the time of the contemplated conception. Though the family history of both husband and wife be ever so good, it is held that if one or both of the parents have acquired undesirable and transmissible characteristics, physical, mental, or moral, then the question of bringing children into the world should be carefully considered, and conscientiously decided, after competent authorities have been consulted concerning the case. The prospective child should always be given the benefit of the doubt in such cases. To bring children into the world merely to gratify personal pleasure or pride, regardless of the welfare of the child, is something utterly unworthy of an intelligent and moral human being.

Fitness for Parenthood.

In determining the "fitness" for parenthood, on the part of husband and wife, the mental, physical, and moral qualities should all be taken into consideration. Weak or abnormal mentality; chronic immorality or perverted moral sense; or diseased or abnormal physical conditions—these should always be regarded as bars to parenthood. To violate this principle is to deliberately violate the fundamental laws of Nature, as well as those principles which are accepted as representing the best thought and customs of the race. A mental, moral, or physical "pervert" or "defective" is manifestly an "unfit," considered as a prospective parent. Parenthood on the part of such individuals is not only a crime against society, but always a base injustice perpetrated upon the offspring.

A very interesting phase of the general subject now before us for consideration is that which touches upon the effect of those particular acquired characteristics which are especially active at the time, or just before the time of conception. The best authorities hold that the influences manifest and active in the prospective father and mother during the period immediately preceding conception will have a marked effect upon the character of the child. The following quotations from authorities on the subject will serve to illustrate this idea.

Riddell says: "The transient physical, mental and moral conditions of the parents, prior to the initial of life, at the time of inception, do affect offspring." Dr. Cowan says: "Through the rightly directed wills of the mother and father, preceding and during ante-natal life, the child's form of body, character of mind, and purity of soul are formed and established. That in its plastic shape, during ante-natal life, like clay in the hand of the potter, it can be molded into absolutely any form of body and soul the parents may knowingly desire." Newton says: "Numerous facts indicate that offspring may be affected and their tendencies shaped by a great variety of influences, among which moods and influences more or less permanent may be included."

Riddell says: "The influence of environmental conditions and pre-natal training are ever evident. Colts from dams that have been under regular training are faster than those from the same mother foaled before she had been trained. The puppies of the trained shepherd dog learn much more rapidly than do those from the untrained animal. No sportsman would think of paying a high price for a puppy, the mother of which was stupid and untrained. The same law applies, only with greater effect, to the human family." Greer says: "No married couple will desire, design and love a babe into existence without the first requisite—good physical health." Grant Allen says: "To prepare ourselves for the duties of maternity and paternity by making ourselves as vigorous and healthful as we can be, is a duty we owe to children unborn." Holbrook says: "It is essential, therefore, that if children are to be well-born, the parents should be careful that at the moment of procreation they are fitted for the performance of so serious an act." Another authority says: "Generation should be preceded by regeneration."

Cowan says: "In the conception of a new life, the mass of mankind observes no law unless it be the law of chance. Out of the licentious or incontinent actions of a husband's nature, conception after a time is discovered to take place. No preparation of body, mind, or soul is made by either parent. Not more than one child in perhaps ten thousand is brought into the world with the consent and loving desire of its parents. The other nine thousand, nine hundred, and ninety nine children are endowed with the accumulated sins of the parents. Is it any wonder that there is so much sin, sickness, drunkenness, suffering, licentiousness, murder, suicide, and premature death, and so little of purity, chastity, success, goodness, happiness and long life in the world?"

Preparation for Parenthood.

The ancient Greeks attached great importance to the mental, moral and physical condition of the parents at the moment of conception, and for a period preceding the same. The Investigations of modern scientists have tended to corroborate the facts upon which the ancient theories were based. Modern science teaches that the life-cells of each parent are impressed with the condition of the respective parents, and retain this impression until they meet and finally coalesce and combine, the combined cell then receiving the result of the original impressions.

The best authorities on the subject claim that a reasonable time of self-restraint and continence should be observed by the prospective parents before the conception of the child. This contention is borne out by the experience of the breeders of fine horses and cattle, who have discovered that the best offspring are produced when the animals have been restrained from sexual intercourse for a reasonable time; this precaution being particularly observed in the case of the male parent animal. Writers on the subject cite a number of instances to prove that this law maintains in human as well is in animal life. It is claimed that Sir Isaac Newton was conceived after a period of over a year of total sexual abstinence on the part of his parents. Many other celebrated men are said to have been conceived after an absence from home on the part of the father, or a temporary absence from home on the part of the mother. Many physicians are able to cite many similar cases observed in the course of their own experience.

The prospective parents should endeavor to bring themselves up to a high degree of physical health and well-being. The blood of the mother should be enriched by proper nutrition, and the organs of the body should be brought to a state of normal functioning along the lines of digestion, assimilation, and elimination.

The minds of both parents should be exercised by reading the right kind of books, and by paying attention to natural objects of interest. A little change of scene will tend to awaken the powers of observation and attention. Riddell says: "If the prospective parents will habitually exercise the reasoning faculties and inventive powers, usually the offspring will have a fair degree of inventive talent and originality, even where these qualities are originally deficient in the parents. When there is a considerable natural talent or where there are latent inventive powers, constant training on the part of the parents will usually give the offspring exceptional powers in this direction."

The prospective parents should also develop and exercise their moral faculties in the period preceding conception. This course will tend to reproduce the same quality in the child. The reverse of this, alas, is also true. A case is cited of a man who procreated a child while plotting a nefarious crime; and the child in after life manifested a tendency toward theft, roguery and rascality, even at a very early age. The lack of moral fibre so often noticed in the sons of rich men who have attained their success through questionable methods is perhaps as much attributable to these pre-conceptual influences as to the "spoiling" environment of the child after birth.

In the period of physical, mental, and moral preparation for parenthood the leading thought of both parents should be: "**Do we wish our child to be like this?**" This thought, if carried as an ideal, will act both in the direction of self-restraint and self-development.

The actual time of the conception of the new life should be carefully chosen, so that it may occur under the best circumstances and conditions. The suggestions embodied in the preceding paragraphs should have been carefully observed; and the time chosen should be one in which a peaceful and happy state of mind is possessed by both parents. The ovum of the woman is believed to have its greatest vitality about the time of the close of each menstrual period, and many good authorities hold that this is not only the natural period for sexual intercourse, but is also the exact period in which the life-forces in the ovum are strongest; and that, consequently, the child conceived at this period is likely to be stronger and more vigorous than the one conceived at a later time between the menstrual periods.

Dr. Stall says: "Medical authorities attach great importance to the mental condition at the moment of conjunction and conception. It is quite universally believed that this is a moment of unparalleled importance to the welfare of the future being. It is an awful crime to beget life carelessly, and when in improper and unworthy mental states. Some people seem to think that the matter of begetting a child, like the matter of selecting a wife, should be left wholly to blind chance. Neither of these two important events can be too much safeguarded by wise and thoughtful consideration. If conception is permitted to take place when either one or both of the parents are in bad health; if the wife is an unwilling mother, and the embryo is developed by her while her whole nature rebels against the admission into the family of a child who is not wanted, the children begotten and born under such circumstances can never be other than sickly, nervous and fretful during their entire childhood, and cross and uncompanionable throughout their whole lives.

"Much of the differences which exist between children of the same parents may be easily attributed to the different bodily and mental conditions of the parents at the period of conjunction, the changed physical, intellectual and emotional states of the parents at the different periods of conception producing the corresponding differences in their offspring. The results of purposed and prepared parenthood are so great and so desirable that a husband and wife should consider these matters carefully, making preparations, and approach the period when they would beget offspring and bring immortal beings into the world with the greatest thoughtfulness, consideration, and also with prayer."

Dr. Hufeland says: "In my opinion, it is of the utmost importance that the moment of conception should be confined to a period when the sensation of collected powers, ardent passion, and a mind cheerful and free from care, invite to it on both sides." Riddell says: "The law of initial impressions is well established. It has been understood and applied by stock-raisers for centuries. Experiments prove that the qualities most highly excited in animals prior to their union are most fully transmitted. The speed of horses and the acquired characters of the dog have been improved by the applications of the law. History and classic literature contain many references that recognize its importance, like Shakespeare's 'Come on, ye cowards; ye were got in fear.' Ancient laws forbade union while parents were intoxicated, because such unions resulted in the production of drunkards and monstrosities. The asylums for the feeble-minded contain hundreds of unfortunate ones that are the product of such unions. The law of initial impressions, like the other laws of heredity, is traced most easily where morbid conditions are transmitted; but fortunately it is quite as potential in the production of desirable qualities. Unusual excitement to the social, intellectual or religious powers on the parents just prior to the inception of the new life frequently produce in the child corresponding tendencies."

Dr. Stockham says: "Many a drunkard owes his lifelong appetite for alcohol to the fact that the inception of his life could be traced to a night of dissipation on the part of his father." Fleming says: "Not only do drunkards transmit to their descendants tendency toward insanity and crime, but even habitually sober parents who at the moment of conception are in a temporary state of drunkenness beget children who are epileptic or paralytic, idiotic or insane, very often microcephalic, or with remarkable weakness of mind, which is transformed at the first favorable occasion into insanity."

The time of conception should undoubtedly be chosen to correspond to a time in which the sex-powers of both parents are at their maximum. This is arrived at by a reasonable period of previous continence and abstinence from sexual relations between the married couple, and by an observance of the natural law which renders the woman most strong sexually at the close of the menstrual period. The husband, as well as the wife, is most strong sexually at this period, as under normal conditions his sex-power is most actively called forth by that of the woman at this period. At this period the wave of sex-power is at its height, and this is the best time for the beginning of the new life. As Riddell says: "Strong, vigorous, chaste sexuality at the time of conception is of supreme importance; it is indispensable to good results. No number of other conditions or factors can be so favorable as to justify the creation of a new life when the vitality of either parent is low. Parents transmit their physical constitution, intellect and morals only to the extent of the sex-power at the time of inception."

It is needless to say that there should exist between the prospective parents a strong bond of affection and attraction. By an irony of civilized life, the term "love child" is applied only to the offspring of unmarried lovers—men and women whose affection or passion have run away with their judgment, and who have "loved not wisely, but too well." Some of the world's greatest men and women have been "love children" of this kind; and in such cases it is probably true that their physical and mental strength has been the result of the ardent feeling animating the parents at the moment of conception. Such children seldom result from the "tired bed" or worn-out passion, love killed by sexual excesses, indifference on the part of one of the participants of the union, "duty" intercourse without affection or passion, or forced sexual relations. Every child should be a "love child" in the true sense of the term. The term should be one of respect, not of reproach. There should be no children but "love children." The fruit of the perfect mating and marriage should be the perfect "love child"—and it would always be so if husbands and wives would but observe the laws of the normal, natural, sex-life.

And, last of all—and perhaps more important than all—is the fact that at the moment of conception the minds and hearts of both of the prospective parents should be united in a strong love and desire for the hoped-for child. At that moment their best natures should blend into each other, and their love for each other fuse into a new love—the love of the child of the union. Under such circumstances, in such act the Cosmic Forces flow unhindered through the beings of the parents, and the new life is begun under the approving smile of Nature.

Maternal Impressions.

One of the oldest and most firmly-rooted beliefs of the race is that which holds that the pregnant mother may, and often does, consciously or unconsciously, impress upon her unborn child certain mental, moral, or physical traits. The majority of persons accept this idea as self-evident, and are able to cite cases within their own personal experience which go to prove the correctness of the popular belief. But certain modern authorities have sought to tear down this belief, and to discredit the general idea. Let us briefly consider both sides of this question.

On the side of the generally accepted belief, Riddell says: "The more I study the influence of maternal impressions upon the life, mentality and character of men, the more I am led to believe that the education and moral training that a child receives before it sees the light of day are the most influential, and, therefore, the most important part of its education." Newton says: "A mother may, during the period of gestation, exercise some influence, by her own voluntary mental and physical action, either unwittingly or purposely, in determining the traits and tendencies of her offspring. This is now a common belief among intelligent people. Every observant teacher could doubtless bear witness to the same general facts, and it would be easy to fill a volume with testimonials from various sources illustrative and confirmatory of the law under discussion. Such facts establish beyond question the conviction that the mother has it largely in her power to confer on her child such a tendency of mind and conformation of brain as shall not only facilitate the acquisition of knowledge in any specific direction, but make it certain that such knowledge will be sought and acquired."

Dr. Fordyce Baker says: "The weight of authority must be conceded to be in favor of the idea that maternal impressions may effect the growth, form and character of a forming child." Dr. Rokitansky says: "The question whether mental emotions do influence the development of the child must be answered 'Yes!'" Dr. Brittain says: "The singular effects produced on the unborn child by the sudden mental emotions of the mother are remarkable examples of a kind of electrotyping on the sensitive surface of living forms. It is doubtless true that the mind's action in such cases may increase or diminish the molecular deposits in the several portions of the system. The precise place which each separate particle assumes may be determined by the influence of thought or feeling. If, for example, there exists in the mother any unusual tendency of the vital forces to the brain at the critical period, there will be a similar cerebral development and activity in the offspring."

Newton says: "The human embryo is formed and developed in all its parts, even to the minutest detail, by and through the action of the vital, mental, and spiritual forces of the mother, which forces act in and through the corresponding portions of her own organism. And while this process may go on unconsciously, or without the mother's voluntary participation or direction, yet she may consciously and purposely so direct her activities as, with a good degree of certainty, to accomplish specifically desired ends in determining the traits and qualities of her offspring." Professor Bayer says: "The influence of the mind of a prospective mother upon her child, before its birth, is of tremendous importance to its active existence as a member of society, from the fact that it lies in the mother's power to shape its mentality, that it may be a power for good or for evil."

The views of that school of thought which is opposed to this old and generally accepted idea of material impressions, are ably presented by Dr. Saleeby, as follows: "Consider the case. The baby is at this time already a baby, though rather small and uncanny, floating in a fluid of its own manufacture. Its sole connection with the mother is by means of its umbilical cord—that is to say, blood-vessels, arterial and venous. There is no nervous connection whatever; absolutely nothing but the blood-stream, carried along a system of tubes. This blood is the child's blood, which it sends forth from itself along the umbillical cord to a special organ, the placenta or afterbirth, half made by itself and half made by the mother, in which the child's blood travels in thin vessels so close to the mother's blood that their contents can be interchanged. Yet the two streams never mix. The child's blood, having disposed of its carbonic acid and waste products to the mother's blood, and having received therefrom oxygen and food, returns so laden to the child. Pray how is the mother's reading of history to make the child a historian? We see now how the learning of geometry on the part of the mother before its birth will not set her baby upon that royal road to geometry of which Euclid rightly denied the existence—any more than after its birth. Such a thing does not happen—**unless we are to call in Telepathy**."

All this argument may seem quite convincing—at first. But when we begin to consider the matter carefully, we begin to perceive the weak places in the argument as above presented. In the first place, it is known that emotions powerfully affect the condition, quality, and "life" of the blood. We know that cheerful emotions impart certain uplifting qualities to the blood, while depressing emotions correspondingly react upon it. Fear, worry, fright, jealousy, etc., are actual poisons to the blood, and have brought on diseased conditions to the persons manifesting these emotions. Moreover, it is known that impaired quality of the blood reacts upon the brain. Is it so unreasonable, then, to hold that emotional states in the mother may react upon the mental and physical condition of the unborn child, through the blood? Does not something similar occur in the case of the babe, after its birth, when it is affected by the conditions of its mother's milk brought on by her depressing emotions, fright, etc.? This would seem to explain at least the matter of emotional reactions between mother and unborn babe.

But the case is not closed with the presentation of the evidence of physiology, important though that may be. There is an entirely different field of science to be drawn upon before the case is closed. The orthodox physiologist makes the mistake of supposing that all mental impulses and transmission of psychic energy require the service of nerves as channels of transmission. While such channels are usually required, we have good reasons for believing that there are exceptions to the rule. There have been found tiny creatures, possessing life and energy, performing the functions of nourishment, elimination, and even of reproduction—and yet without a nervous system. In one well-known instance, that of the moneron, we find not only an absence of a nervous system but also the lack of organs of any kind—and yet the creature lives, acts, moves, eats, thinks, and reproduces itself.

Then, again, consider the moving cells of the blood, unconnected with the brain, unattached to the nervous system, and yet rushing to the work of repairing a wound, or of repelling an intruding germ, in obedience to a mental command from the controlling subconscious mental regions of the living creature. How does the mental impulse reach these cells and others of similar nature in the system? If we were not so sure of the facts, might we not feel inclined to say with Dr. Saleeby, in the above quoted sentence: "Such a thing does not happen—unless we are to call in telepathy."

Moreover, examining Dr. Saleeby's statement, we see mention made of the placenta at being "half made by the embryo, and half made by the mother." How does this co-operation and co-ordination of effort and subconscious will arise? How does the subconscious mentality of the embryo know that the subconscious mentality of the mother is making its half of the placenta, or vice versa? Again, how is the subconscious mentality of the mother affected by the presence and development of the child—how do her mammary glands respond to the growth and development of the child? In short, how is the manifest co-operation and co-ordination between the "nature" of the mother and the "nature" of the child possible, unless there exists some psychical, as well as some physical, relation between the two beings.

The person conscientiously considering this subject must include in his thought the discoveries of modern psychology concerning what is known as the "subconscious mind," which controls the unconscious and instinctive functions of the physical body, and also receives impressions and suggestions from the surface consciousness of its owner. This factor being admitted to our thought on the subject, we may find it possible to accept the idea of material impressions from mother to child operating from the subconscious mind of the mother to that of the child. In other words, that there is a subconscious mental connection, as well as the physical connection, between the mother and her unborn child.

Many careful thinkers (and observers) find it just as easy to accept the fact of this strange "sympathetic co-ordination" between a mother and her unborn child as it is to accept the very frequent "sympathetic sickness" of the husband during the pregnancy of his wife—or of the "sympathetic labor pains" so often experienced by the husband during the confinement of his wife. Both of the latter two cases occur too often to permit the phenomenon to be denied off hand by those who would set aside all facts not agreeing with their particular personal theories. There is no nervous system connecting husband and wife, and of such cases the critic like Dr. Saleeby might say: "Such a thing does not happen—**unless we call in telepathy**!"

The fact remains that many things actually happen which according to the orthodox physiological theories "**cannot** happen." But they DO happen, nevertheless, whether we call it "telepathy" or merely label it "certain facts, the exact causes of which Science in the present state of its knowledge (or ignorance) cannot definitely determine." One irrefutable fact outweighs a ton of mere general denials of possibility.

It is recorded that the mother of Charles Kingsley believed in maternal impressions, and during her period of pregnancy exercised her imagination and emotions in the direction of wishing, and imagining, that the coming child should have the same love of Devonshire scenery that so delighted her. The result proved her theory, for though Kingsley never saw Devonshire until he was a man of thirty years of age, every Devonshire scene had a mysterious charm for him throughout his entire life. It is said that Robert Burns was so strongly impressed parentally by the old Scotch songs and ballads that his mother sung during her pregnancy, that his whole nature longed to express itself in like measure and substance. He always believed that his poetic spirit was kindled by this tendency on the part of his mother during the period preceding his birth.

The mother of Napoleon Bonaparte during several months of her pregnancy, accompanied her husband during his military campaigns in Corsica, and during the entire term she lived in an atmosphere of battles, military strategy, and troops. When the boy was very young he manifested an unusual interest in war and conquest, and his whole mind had the military bent, although his brothers were in no wise remarkable in this direction. The artist, Flaxman, stated that his mother had related to him how for several months prior to his birth she had spent many hours each day studying drawings and engravings, and endeavoring to visualize by memory the beautiful figures of the human body drawn by the masters. The result was that from early childhood Flaxman manifested an intense delight in drawing; and in after life his drawings were regarded as masterpieces. He, and his mother, always attributed his talent to the parental impressions above mentioned.

"Buffalo Bill" was believed to owe his characteristics to the mental states of his mother, the family living in Missouri during the days of frontier fights and disturbances, the mother being called upon several times to exercise resourceful courage and fortitude. A well-known worker along the lines of liberal Christianity is said to have attributed his tendencies in that direction to the prayers of his mother, during her pregnancy, that the child might be true to the teachings of the Christ, and should be a laborer in the cause of human brotherhood. This man, relating the fact, said: "I may have been converted before I was born." A well-known writer along the lines of moral philosophy is believed by friends to owe his talent to the earnest thoughts and hopes of his mother during pregnancy—she is said to have pictured the child as a son destined to become a great moral philosopher, her mind being so firmly fixed on this fact that she felt it was already an assured fact.

The Greeks were wont to surround the pregnant women with beautiful statuary, and it is recorded that in many cases the children afterward born closely resembled these works of art and beauty. It is claimed that many Italian women closely resemble the face shown in Raphael's "Madonna," copies of this celebrated picture being quite common in Italian households. Frances Willard, the temperance worker, is said to have very closely resembled a young woman of whom her mother was very fond. Many family resemblances are believed to have arisen in this way, rather than by heredity. Zerah Colburn, the mathematical prodigy whose feats astounded the scientific world in the early part of the last century, is said to have derived his wonderful faculty from maternal impressions of this kind; his mother is said to have occupied much of her time during her pregnancy in studying arithmetic and working problems, the study being quite new to her and proving very interesting.

Cases similar to those above quoted might be duplicated almost indefinitely. The story is practically the same in each and every case. The principle involved is always that the pregnant mother took a decided interest in certain subjects, studies, and work, and that the child when born manifested at an early age similar tastes and inclinations. But far more important to the average prospective parent is the fact that many authorities positively claim that **any pregnant mother may consciously and deliberately influence and shape the character, physical, mental, and moral of her unborn child**.

Newton well says, on this subject: "In the cases usually given to the public bearing on this topic, the moulding power appears to have been exercised merely by accident or chance; that is, without any intelligent purpose on the part of mothers to produce the results. Can there be any doubt that similar means, if purposely and wisely adopted, and applied with the greater care and precision which enlightened intention secure, would produce under the same law even more perfect results. Is it not altogether probable that an intentional direction of the vital or mental forces to any particular portion of the brain will cause a development and activity in the corresponding portion of the brain of the offspring? There seems to be no reasonable ground on which these propositions can be denied. The brain is made up of a congeries of organs which are the organs of distinct faculties of the mind or soul. It follows, then, that if the mother during gestation maintains a special activity of any one brain organ, or group of organs, in her brain, she thereby causes more development of the corresponding organ or group in the brain of the fetus. She thus determines a tendency in the child to special activity of the faculties, of which such organs are the instruments. It is plain, furthermore, that if any one organ or faculty may thus be cultivated before birth, and its activity enhanced for life, so may any other—and so may all. It would seem, then, clearly within the bounds of possibility that a mother, by pursuing a systematic and comprehensive method, may give a well-rounded and harmoniously developed organism to her child—notwithstanding her own defects, which, under the unguided operation of hereditary law, are likely to be repeated in her offspring. Or it is within her power to impart a leading tendency in any specific direction that she may deem desirable, for a life of the highest usefulness. **In this way ancestral defects and undesirable hereditary traits, of whatever nature or however strong, may be overcome, or in a good degree counterbalanced by giving greater activity to counteracting tendencies**; and, in this way, too, it would appear the coveted gifts of genius may be conferred. In other words, it would seem to be within the mother's power, by the voluntary and intelligent direction of her own forces, in orderly and systematic methods, both to mold the physical form to lines of beauty, and shape the mental, moral, and spiritual features of her child to an extent to which no limit can be assigned."

I think that in the pages of this particular part of the book the prospective parent may find hints and general directions toward a clearly defined ideal, which is carefully studied, and as carefully put into practice will produce results far beyond the dreams of the average man and woman. The hope is a magnificent one, and the best testimony is in favor of the possibility of its actual realization.

LESSON VIII
EUGENICS AND CHARACTER

The rapidly growing interest in Eugenics, and the scientific consideration of the world-wide decline in the birth-rate have drawn attention to the study of the eugenic factors which determine the production of high ability in offspring. Many distinguished investigators have conducted long and exhaustive investigations for the purpose of ascertaining and summarizing all possible biological data concerning the parentage and birth of the most notable persons born in European countries, and to a lesser extent in America.

The investigations are now acquiring a fresh importance, because, while it is becoming recognized that we are gaining a control over the conditions of birth, the production of children has itself gained an importance. The world is no longer to be bombarded by an exuberant stream of babies, good, bad, and indifferent in quality, with mankind to look on calmly at the struggle for existence among them. Whether we like it or not, the quantity is steadily diminishing, and the question of quality is beginning to assume a supreme significance. The question then is being anxiously asked: "What are the conditions which assure the finest quality in our children?"

A German scientist, Dr. Vaerting, of Berlin, published just before the War a treatise on the subject of the most favorable age in parents for the production of offspring of ability. He treated the question in an entirely new spirit, not merely as a matter of academic discussion, but rather as a practical matter of vital importance to the welfare of modern society. He starts by asserting that "our century has been called the century of the child," and that for the child all manner of rights are now being claimed. But, he wisely adds, there is seldom considered the prime right of all the child's rights, i. e., the right of the child to the best ability and capacity for efficiency that his parents are able to transmit to him. The good doctor adds that this right is the root of all children's rights; and that when the mysteries of procreation have been so far revealed as to enable this right to be won, we shall, at the same time renew the spiritual aspect of the nations.

The writer referred to decided that the most easily ascertainable and measurable factor in the production of ability, and efficiency in offspring, and a factor of the greatest significance, is the age of the parents at the child's birth. He investigated a number of cases of men of ability and efficiency, along these lines, and made a careful summary of his results. Some of his results are somewhat startling, and may possibly require the corroboration of other investigators before they can be accepted as authoritative; but they are worthy of being carefully considered at the present time, pending such further investigation.

Vaerting found that the fathers who were themselves not notably intellectual have a decidedly more prolonged power of procreating distinguished children than is possessed by distinguished fathers. The former may become the fathers of eminent children from the period of sexual maturity up to the age of forty-three or beyond. When, however, the father is himself of high intellectual distinction, the records show that he was nearly always under thirty, and usually under twenty-five years of age at the time of the birth of his distinguished son, although the proportion of youthful fathers in the general population is relatively small. The eleven youngest fathers on Vaerting's list, from twenty-one to twenty-five years of age, were with one exception themselves more or less distinguished; while the fifteen oldest, from thirty-nine to sixty years of age, were all without exception undistinguished.

Among the sons on the latter list are to be found much greater names (such as Goethe, Bach, Kant, Bismarck, Wagner, etc.) than are to be found among the sons of young and more distinguished fathers, for here is only one name (Frederick the Great) of the same caliber. The elderly fathers belonged to the large cities, and were mostly married to wives very much younger than themselves. Vaerting notes that the most eminent men have frequently been the sons of fathers who were not engaged in intellectual avocations at all, but earned their living as humble craftsmen. He draws the conclusion from these data that strenuous intellectual energy is much more unfavorable than hard physical labor to the production of marked ability in the offspring. Intellectual workers, therefore, he argues, must have their children when young, and we must so modify our social ideals and economic conditions as to render this possible.

Vaerting, however, holds that the mother need not be equally young; he finds some superiority, indeed, provided the father is young, in somewhat elderly mothers, and there were no mothers under twenty-three on the list. The rarity of genius among the offspring of distinguished parents he attributes to the unfortunate tendency to marry too late; and he finds that the distinguished men who marry late rarely have any children at all. Speaking generally, and apart from the production of genius, he holds that women have children too early, before their psychic development is completed, while men have children too late, when they have already "in the years of their highest psychic generative fitness planted their most precious seed in the mud of the street."

The eldest child was found to have by far the best chance of turning out distinguished, and in this fact Vaerting finds further proof of his argument. The third son has the next best chance, and then the second, the comparatively bad position of the second being attributed to the too brief interval which often follows the birth of the first child. He also notes that of all the professions the clergy come beyond comparison first as the parents of distinguished sons (who are, however, rarely of the highest degree of eminence), lawyers following, while officers in the army and physicians scarcely figure at all. Vaerting is inclined to see in this order, especially in the predominance of the clergy, the favorable influence of an unexhausted reserve of energy and a habit of chastity on intellectual procreativeness.

It should be remembered, however, that Vaerting's cases on his list were all those of Germans, and, therefore, the influence of the characteristic social customs and conditions of the German people must be taken into account in the consideration.

Havelock Ellis in his well known work "Study of British Genius" dealt on a still larger scale, and with a somewhat more precise method, with many of the same questions as illustrated by British cases. After the publication of Vaerting's work, Ellis re-examined his cases, and rearranged his data. His results, like those of the German authority, showed a special tendency for genius to appear in the eldest child, though there was no indication of notably early marriage in the parents. He also found a similar predominance of the clergy among the fathers, and a similar deficiency of army officers and physicians.

Ellis found that the most frequent age of the father was thirty-two years, but that the average age of the father at the distinguished child's birth was 36.6 years; and that when the fathers were themselves distinguished their age was not, as Vaerting found in Germany, notably low at the birth of their distinguished sons, but higher than the general average, being 37.5 years. He found fifteen distinguished sons of distinguished British fathers, but instead of being nearly always under thirty and usually under twenty-five, as Vaerting found it in Germany, the British distinguished father has only five times been under thirty, and among these only twice under twenty-five. Moreover, precisely the most distinguished of the sons (Francis Bacon and William Pitt) had the oldest fathers, and the least distinguished sons the youngest fathers.

Ellis says of his general conclusions resulting from this investigation: "I made some attempts to ascertain whether different kinds of genius tend to be produced by fathers who were at different periods of life. I refrained from publishing the results as I doubted whether the numbers dealt with were sufficiently large to carry any weight. It may, however, be worth while to record them, as possibly they are significant. I made four classes of men of genius: (1) Men of Religion, (2) Poets, (3) Practical Men, (4) Scientific Men and Sceptics. (It must not, of course, be supposed that in this last group all the scientific men were sceptics, or all the sceptics scientific.) The average age of the fathers at the distinguished son's birth was, in the first group, 35 years; in the second and third group, 37 years; and in the last group, 40 years. (It may be noted, however, that the youngest father of all the history of British genius, aged sixteen, produced Napier, who introduced logarithms.)

"It is difficult not to believe that as regards, at all events, the two most discrepant groups, the first and last, we come upon a significant indication. It is not unreasonable to suppose that in the production of men of religion in whose activity emotion is so potent a factor, the youthful age of the father should prove favorable; while for the production of genius of a more coldly intellectual and analytic type more elderly fathers are demanded. If that should prove to be so, it would become a source of happiness to religious parents to have their children early, while irreligious parents should be advised to delay parentage.

"It is scarcely necessary to remark that the age of the mothers is probably quite as influential as that of the fathers. Concerning the mothers, however, we always have less precise information. My records, so far as they go, agree with Vaerting's for German genius, in indicating that an elderly mother is more likely to produce a child of genius than a very youthful mother. There were only fifteen mothers recorded under twenty-five years of age, while thirteen were over thirty-nine years; the most important age for mothers was twenty-seven.

"On all these points we certainly need controlling evidence from other countries. Thus, before we insist with Vaerting that an elderly mother is a factor in the production of genius, we may recall that even in Germany the mothers of Goethe and Nietzsche were both eighteen at their distinguished son's birth. A rule which permits of such tremendous exceptions scarcely seems to bear the strain of emphasis."

The student, however, must always remember that while the study of genius and exceptionable talent is highly interesting, and even, as is quite probable, not without significance for the general laws of heredity, still we must beware of too hastily drawing conclusions from it to bear on the practical questions of eugenics. Genius is rare—and, in a certain sense, abnormal. Laws meant for application to the general population must be based on a study of the general population. Vaerting, himself, realized how inadequate it was to confine our study to cases of genius.

Another investigator, Marro, an Italian scientist, in his well-known book on puberty which was published several years ago, brought forth some interesting data showing the result of the age of the parents on the moral and intellectual characters of school-children in Northern Italy. He found that children with fathers below twenty-six at their birth showed the maximum of bad conduct and the minimum of good; they also yielded the greatest proportion of children of irregular, troublesome, or lazy character, but not of really perverse children—the latter being equally distributed among fathers of all ages. The largest number of cheerful children belonged to the young fathers, while the children tended to become more melancholy with ascending age of the fathers. Young fathers produced the largest number of intelligent, as well as of troublesome children; but when the very exceptional intelligent children were considered separately, they were found to be more usually the offspring of elderly fathers.

As regarded the mothers, Marro found that the children of young mothers (under twenty-one) are superior, both as regards conduct and intelligence, though the more exceptionally intelligent children tended to belong to more mature mothers. When the parents were both in the same age-groups, the immature and the elderly groups tended to produce more children who were unsatisfactory, both as regards conduct and intelligence—the intermediate group yielding the most satisfactory results of this kind.

Havelock Ellis makes the following plea for further investigations along these lines, in the interest of the well-being of the race: "But we have need of inquiries made on a more wholesale and systematic scale. They are no longer of a merely speculative character. We no longer regard children as the 'gifts of God' flung into our helpless hands; we are beginning to realize that the responsibility is ours to see that they come into the world under the best conditions, and at the moments when their parents are best fitted to produce them. Vaerting proposes that it should be the business of all school authorities to register the ages of the pupils' parents. This is scarcely a provision to which even the most susceptible parent could reasonably object, though there is no cause to make the declaration compulsory where a 'conscientious' objection existed, and in any case the declaration would not be public.

"It would be an advantage—although this might be more difficult to obtain —to have the date of the children's marriage, and of the birth of previous children, as well as some record of the father's standing in his occupation. But even the ages of the parents alone would teach us much when correlated with the school position of the pupil in intelligence and conduct. It is quite true that there are unavoidable fallacies. We are not, as in the case of genius, dealing with people whose life-work is complete and open to the whole world's examination.

"The good and clever child is not necessarily the forerunner of the first-class man or woman; and many capable and successful men have been careless in attendance at lectures, and rebellious to discipline. Moreover, the prejudice and limitations of the teachers have to be recognized. Yet when we are dealing with millions most of these fallacies would be smoothed out. We should be, once for all, in a position to determine authoritatively the exact bearing of one of the simplest and most vital factors of the betterment of the race. We should be in possession of a new clue to guide us in the creation of the man in the coming world. Why not begin today?"

Considerable attention on the part of the American thinking public has been directed toward the investigations and researches of Casper L. Redfield. Mr. Redfield combats the orthodox scientific position that the acquired qualities are not transmitted to offspring; and he most positively states that such characteristics are transmitted to offspring, and are really the causes which have tended toward the evolution and progress of the race. But he insists upon this vital point, namely, that the parent must already have acquired improved quality before he can transmit improvement to the offspring—and that before he can have acquired this improved quality, he must have lived sufficiently long to have experienced the causes which have developed improvement in himself. Consequently, he holds that **delayed parentage produces great men**.

Mr. Redfield several years ago offered a prize of two hundred dollars to anyone who could show that a single one of the great men of history was the product of a succession of young parents, or was produced by a line of ancestry represented by more than three generations to a century. But no one ever claimed the prize money. According to Mr. Redfield's doctrine, race improvement is and will be accomplished as the result of effort, physical and mental, upon the part of prospective parents, particularly if the period of effort is sustained over a considerable number of years previous to reproduction.

The following quotations from Mr. Redfield's writing will give a general idea of his lines of thought and his theories. He says:

"At some time in the past there was a common ancestor for man and the ape. At that time the mental ability of the man was the same as that of the ape, because at that time man and the ape were the same person. From that common ancestor there have been derived two main lines of descent, one leading to man and the other to the ape of today. In the line leading to man, mental ability has increased little by little so that today the mental ability of the man is far above that of the ape. While it may not be literally true for each and every generation between that common ancestor and man of the present time, still we will commit no error if we divide the total increase in mental ability by the number of intervening generations and say that each generation in turn was a little superior to that which produced it. Now it happens that mental ability is something which is inherited—is transmitted from parent to offspring. Take that fact with the fact that there has been a regular (or irregular) increase in mental ability in the generations leading to man, and it will be seen that each generation in succession transmitted to its offspring more than it inherited from its parents. **But a parent cannot transmit something which he did not have.** Where and how did those generations get that ability which they transmitted but did not inherit?"

Mr. Redfield in his writings shows that what is true of the human race is true of high-bred domesticated animals, namely, the cow of high milk producing breeds; the fast running and trotting horses; and the highly developed hunting dogs. To each case he applies his question: "Where and how did those generations of animals get that power which they transmitted but did not inherit?" In his investigations he claims to have discovered the secret, namely, that the ancestors, throughout several generations, had each acquired the power which it transmitted, which added to the inherited power raised the general power of the stock. This arose from careful breeding, and directly from the fact that the average age of the parent was much higher in the highly-bred stock than in the "scrub" or ordinary run of stock. In other words, **delayed parentage produced better offspring**.

Mr. Redfield proceeds to argue from these facts as follows: "At one time man and ape reproduced at the same average age, whereas now they reproduce at widely different ages. Going back to the time when man and ape separated, our ancestors survived by physical and mental activity in securing food and escaping from enemies. As time went on man reproduced at later and later average age until now he reproduces at about thirty years from birth of parent to birth of offspring. When time between generations stretched out in the man line more than it did in the ape line, the man acquired **more mental development before he reproduced** than did the ape, and he did this because he was mentally active more years before reproducing. The successive generations leading to modern man transmitted to offspring more than they inherited from their parents, and the generations which did this are the same generations which acquired, before reproducing, the identical thing which they transmitted in excess of inheriting.

"Coming now to those rare men of whom we have only a few in a century, how were they produced? It should be noted that each one had two parents, four grandparents, and eight great-grandparents. Also that they are certainly improvements over their great-grandparents. If they were not such improvements, then there would be many 'rare' cases in a century. In looking into the pedigrees of these great men it is found that they were sons of parents of nearly all ages, but were predominantly sons of elderly parents. While we sometimes find comparatively young parents in the pedigree of a great man, we never find a succession of young parents. Neither do we find an intellectually great man produced by a pedigree extending over three generations. The great man is produced only when the average for three generations is on the elderly side of what is normal. The average age of one thousand fathers, grandfathers, and great-grandfathers in the pedigrees of eminent men was found to be over forty years. Great men rise from ordinary stock only when several generations in succession acquire mental efforts in excess amounts before reproducing."

It is the opinion of the present writer that the theories of Mr. Redfield are in the main true, and that in the future much valuable information will be obtained along the same lines, which will tend to corroborate his general conclusions. One's attention needs but to be plainly directed to the matter, and then he will see that it is absurd to think of a creature transmitting to his offspring qualities which neither he or his mate had inherited or acquired. If there were no transmission of acquired qualities there would be no improvement—and in fact, we know that the bulk of inherited qualities were at some time in the history of the race "acquired." And, reasoning along the same line, we may see that the young parents who have not had as yet an opportunity to acquire mental power cannot expect to transmit it to their offspring—all that they can do is to transmit the inherited stock qualities plus the small acquired power which they have gained in their limited experience. And, finally, it is seen that offspring produced at a riper age of parenthood, continued over several generations, tend toward unusual ability and powers. Consequently, the people or nation with a higher average age of parenthood may logically expect to attain greater mental powers than the peoples lacking that quality. And what is true of a people or nation is of course true of a particular family.

The subject touched upon in this part of our book is one of the greatest interest to careful students of Eugenics; and is one which calls for careful and unprejudiced consideration from all persons having the interest of the race at heart.

LESSON IX
THE DETERMINATION OF SEX

The term "The Determination of Sex" is employed in two general senses in scientific circles.

The first usage is that of the biologist, and it includes within its scope merely the discovery and understanding of the **causes** which determine whether the embryo shall develop into a male or into a female. In the discussion of the subject from this standpoint there is but little, if any, attention given to the question of whether the sex of the unborn child may be determined by methods under the control of man. The biologist simply studies the causes which seem to lead to the production of an individual of one or the other sex, without regard to whether these causes, when discovered, may or may not be amendable to human control.

An authority, speaking of this standpoint concerning the question referred to, says: "We may discover the causes of storms or earthquakes, and when our knowledge of them is sufficiently advanced we may be able to predict them as successfully as astronomers predict eclipses, but there is little hope that we shall ever be able to control them. So it may be with sex; a complete understanding of the causes which determine it may not necessarily give us the power of producing one or the other sex at will, or even of predicting the sex in any given case. Whether we shall ever be able to influence the causes of sex-determination cannot as yet be foretold; at present, biologists are engaged in the less practical, but immensely interesting, problem, of discovering what those causes are."

The second usage of the term, includes and embraces the idea of the voluntary determination or control of the sex of the future child, by means of certain methods or certain systems of treatment, etc. Of recent years, science has been devoting considerable attention to the question of whether or not man may not be able to produce any particular sex at will, by means of certain systems or methods of procedure. Many theories have been evolved, and many plans and methods have been advocated, often with the expenditure of much energy and enthusiasm on the part of the promulgators and their adherents.

In this lesson there will be briefly presented to you the general consensus of modern thought on the subject, with a general outline of the favorite methods and systems advocated by the several schools of thought concerned in the investigation.

Professor Doncaster, the well-known authority on the subject, says: "But little progress has been made in the direction of predicting the sex of any child, and, if possible, even less in artificially influencing the determination of its sex. When the general principles arrived at are borne in mind, it must be confessed that the prospects of our ever attaining this power of control or even of prediction are not very hopeful, but the possibility of it cannot be yet regarded as entirely excluded. The general conclusions arrived at are that sex is determined by a physiological condition of the embryonic cells, that this condition is induced, at least in the absence of disturbing causes, by the presence of a particular sex-chromosome. [A "chromosome" is a portion of the chromatin, or substance characteristic of the nucleus of the cell, this nucleus seemingly controlling the life-processes of the cell.] But there is evidence, which for the present at least cannot be neglected, that certain extraneous conditions acting on the egg or early embryo may perhaps be able to counteract the effect of sex chromosome.

"Quite generally, then, there are two conceivable methods by which the sex might be artificially influenced in any particular case; firstly, if means could be found of ensuring that any particular fertilized ovum received the required chromosomes; and, secondly, by the discovery of methods which always effect the ovum or embryo in such a way as to produce the desired sex. Many suggestions for applying both methods have been made, some of which have attained considerable notoriety, but hitherto none of them has stood the test of practical experience. In the case of the higher animals, especially of the mammals, in which the embryo develops in the maternal uterus until long after the sex is irrevocably decided, it is obviously difficult to apply methods which might influence the sex after fertilization, even if it were certainly known that such methods were ever really effective.

"Apart from the few experiments like those of Hertwig on rearing tadpoles at different temperatures, there have been a very few cases in which there is even a suggestion that the sex of the fertilized egg can be modified by environment, and the belief that this is possible has been entirely abandoned by many of the leading investigators of the subject. It is probable, therefore, that if it will ever be possible to predict or determine artificially the sex of a particular child, the means will have to be sought in some method of influencing the output of germ-cells in such a way that one kind is produced rather than the other. It is in this way that Heape and others interpret the results of their investigations; they find that certain conditions affect the sex-ratio of cells, and they explain the result by assuming that **under some circumstances male-determining ova are produced in excess, and under other circumstances, female-determining**."

Professor Rumley Dawson holds to the opinion that the male-determining and female-determining ova are discharged alternately from the ovaries. In woman one ovum is usually discharged each month, and it is maintained that on one month the ovum is male-determining, and in the next, female-determining. It is obvious that exceptions must occur, for boy and girl twins are quite common, but if the cases which support the hypothesis are taken by themselves, and the exceptions explained away, it is possible to make out a strong case in favor of this theory. Some authorities hold that the right ovary produces male-determining ova, and the left ovary female-determining, and that the two ovaries discharge an ovum alternately, but an impartial examination of the evidence for this belief shows that it rests on very slender foundations. Experiments on the lower animals have shown that after the complete removal of one ovary the female may produce young of both sexes. Women, also, have produced children of a particular sex after the corresponding ovary has been removed, and it is hardly possible to believe that the removal in all these cases was incomplete. On the whole it must be concluded that the theory is insufficiently supported by the evidence.

Another widely promulgated and vigorously supported theory is that which holds that the sex of the future child may be determined by specific nutrition of the mother before conception, and in some cases after conception. Schenk's theory, advanced about 1900, attracted much attention at the time. He based his method on the observation that a number of women whose children were all girls all excreted sugar in their urine, such as happens in the case of persons affected with diabetes. From this he suspected that the physiological condition which leads to the excretion of sugar was inimical to the development of male-determining ova, and that males could be produced by its prevention. He therefore recommended that those who desire a male child should undergo treatment similar to that prescribed for diabetes for two or three months before conception, and held that a boy would be produced by these methods. Although this method has had considerable vogue, it cannot be held to have been established on a scientific basis.

Doncaster says "The general conclusion with regard to man must therefore be that if sex is determined solely by the spermatozoon there is no hope either of influencing or predicting it in special cases. On the other hand, there is considerable evidence that the ovum has some share in the effect, and if this is so, before any practical results are reached it will be necessary to discover which of two conceivable causes of sex-determination is the true one. It is possible that there are two kinds of ova, as well as two kinds of spermatozoa, and that there is a selective fertilization of such a kind that one kind of spermatozoon only fertilizes one kind of ovum, the second kind of spermatozoon the second kind of ovum. If this should prove to be the case, it is possible that means might be found of influencing or predicting that kind of ovum which is discharged under any set of conditions. Secondly, it is possible that the ova are potentially all alike, but that their physiological condition may under some circumstances be so altered that the sex is determined independently of the spermatozoon. * * * It is hardly possible to avoid the conclusion that the sex of the offspring may be influenced, at least under certain circumstances, by the mother. The search for means of influencing the sex of the offspring through the mother is not of necessity doomed to failure. No results of a really positive kind have been obtained hitherto, and some of the facts point so clearly to sex-determination by the male germ-cell alone in man and other animals that many investigators have concluded that the quest is hopeless; but until an adequate explanation has been given of certain phenomena discovered in the investigation of the subject, it seems more reasonable to maintain an open mind, and to regard the control of sex in man as an achievement not entirely impossible of realization."

Another writer on the subject has said: "Every individual among the higher animals, whether male or female, begins as an impregnated ovum in the mother's body. Any such ovum contains elements of constitution from both of its parents. In the earliest existence of this impregnated ovum, there is a season of sexual indifference, or indecision, in which the embryo is both male and female, having the characteristic rudiments of each sex, only indifferently manifested. In this stage, the embryo is susceptible of being influenced by external conditions to develop more strongly in the one or the other direction and thus become distinctly and permanently male or female. It is evident that this is the season in the development of the individual in which influencing conditions and causes must operate in deciding its sex, although it is possible in some of the lower animals to alter the tendency of sex in the embryo from one sex to the other, even after it has been quite definitely determined. It is well established, in fact, that differences do not come from a difference in the ova themselves; that is, there is not one kind of ova from the female which becomes female, while other ova become male, for it is possible to alter the tendency toward the one sex or the other after the ovum has been fertilized and the embryo has begun its career of development. This possible change in sex tendency in the embryo also proves that sex is not decided by a difference in the spermatozoa; that is some of the sperm cells from the father are not male, while others are female, in their constitution.

"It is incorrect to suppose, as has been held by some theorists, that one testicle give rise to male spermatozoa and the other to female spermatozoa, for both male and female offspring have been produced from the same male parent after one testicle or the other has been removed. The same is true in cases in which either ovary has been removed from the mother; that is, male and female offspring are produced from mothers in whom either ovary has been removed. In like manner, the sex of offspring is shown not to be materially affected by the comparative vigor of the parents; thus, a stronger father than mother does not necessarily produce one sex to the exclusion of the other. These negative decisions are important because they simplify the solution of the problem of sex-determination, by excluding, more or less fully, various causes which have been supposed to operate quite forcibly in deciding the sex of offspring. Some of the more positive agencies that enter into the determination of sex are found (1) in the influence of nutrition upon the embryo during its indifferent stage of sexual development, and (2) in the constitution and general condition of the mother before and during the early stages of pregnancy. These two factors appear to enter more fully than any others in the decision of the sex in offspring, and deserve the greatest consideration. The influence of food in supplying the embryo with nourishment for its development is, perhaps, the most potent of these determining causes."

Investigators along the line of theory indicated in the above last quotation, i. e., the theory of sex determination by means of nourishment of the mother and embryo, have presented a volume of reports which demand respectful consideration. The general report may be said to be the discovery that **abundant nourishment during the period of sexual neutrality tends to produce females; while lack of abundant nutrition during such period tends to produce males**.

These experiments, of course, have been chiefly performed upon the lower animals. The frog has been a favorite subject of such experiments—the tadpole stage being the one selected, because in that stage there exists a lack of sex, the stage being one of sex neutrality. Professor Yung's celebrated experiments will illustrate this class of experiments. Here were chosen 300 tadpoles, which when left to themselves manifested a ratio of 57 prospective females to 43 prospective males. These were divided into three classes of 100 tadpoles each. Each class was then fed upon one of several kinds of nutritious diet in order to ascertain the change in sex-tendency due to such food. The first set, with an original ratio of femaleness of 54 to 46, were fed abundantly on beef, and the ratio of femaleness was changed to 78 to 22. The second class, with a ratio of femaleness of 61 to 39, were fed on fish (specially nourishing to frogs), and the ratio changed to 81 to 19. The third class, with a ratio of 56 to 44, were fed upon a still more nutritious diet (i. e., that of frogs' flesh), and the ratio was raised to 92 to 8. In short, the experiments showed that the increase of nourishment in diet changed every two out of three male-tendency tadpoles into females. The experiment was held to prove that a rich diet, affording nourishment, during the period of sexual neutrality in the embryo, tended to develop femaleness.

The advocates of this theory also point to the instance of the bees. With the bees, the larva of ordinary worker-bees are fed ordinary food, and do not develop sex; while the larva which is intended to produce the queen-bee is fed specially nutritious "royal food," and consequently develops larger size and full female sex powers. If the queen is killed, or dies, the hive of bees proceeds to produce a new queen by means of feeding a selected larva with the "royal food" and thus developing full femaleness in it. It is said by some authorities that in cases in which some other of the larva accidently receive, through mistake, crumbs of the "royal food," they, too, grow to an extraordinary size, and develop fertility. This fact is held by the advocates of the nutrition theory to go toward establishing the fact that abundant nourishment of the embryo, during the neutral stage, tends to produce femaleness in it. They also claim that caterpillars which are very poorly nourished before entering into the chrysalis stage usually develop into male butterflies, while those highly nourished in the said stage tend to become females. Experiments on sheep have shown that when the ewes are particularly well nourished the offspring will show a large proportion of females.

A writer, favoring the theory in question, says: "In general, it is reasonable to infer that the higher sexual organization which constitutes the female is to be attained in the greatest number of cases by embryos which have superior vital conditions during the formative period. Among human beings, some facts of general observation become significant in the light of the foregoing inferences. After epidemics, after wars, after seasons of privation and distress, the tendency is toward a majority of male births. On the other hand, abundant crops, low prices, peace, contentment and prosperity tend to increase the number of females born. Mothers in prosperous families usually have more girls; mothers in families of distress have more boys. Large, well-fed, fully developed, healthy women, who are of contented and passive disposition, generally become mothers of families abounding in girls; while mothers who are small or spare of flesh, who are poorly fed, restless, unhappy, overworked, exhausted by frequent childbearing, or who are reduced by other causes which waste their vital energies, usually give birth to a greater number of boys. As a general proposition, the facts and inferences tend to establish the truth of the doctrine with women, that, the more favorable the vital conditions of the mother during the period in which the sex of her offspring is being determined, the greater the ratio of females she will bear; the less favorable her vital conditions at such times, the greater will be her tendency to bear males. That many apparent exceptions occur does not disprove the general tendency here maintained. Moreover, it is impossible to know in all cases what were the conditions of the mother's organism at the time in which her child was in its delicate balance between predominant femaleness and maleness; else many cases which seemingly disprove the proposition would be found to be forcible illustrations of its truth. Still further, it is probable that other causes besides those here mentioned act with greater or less effect in determining the sex of offspring."

Based upon this general theory of the relation of nutrition to sex-determination, many methods and systems have been devised by as many authorities, and have been followed and promulgated by as many schools. Without going into the almost endless detail which would be necessitated by a synopsis of these various methods and systems, it may be said that they all consist of plans having for their object the decrease of nutrition of the woman in cases in which male children are desired, and the increase of nutrition in cases in which female children are sought for. This increase or decrease in nutrition is enforced for a reasonable period before the time selected for the conception of the child, and also for a reasonable period after the time of conception. The decrease in nutrition does not consist of "starvation," but rather of a "training diet" similar to that followed by athletics, and from which dietary all rich foods, sweets, etc., are absent. In fact, the average dietary advocated by the "Eat and Grow Thin" writers would seem to be almost identical with that of the "male offspring" theorists.

Many persons who have followed the methods and systems based on the nutrition theory above mentioned claim to have been more or less successful in the production of the particular sex desired, but many exceptions to the rule are noted, and some writers on the subject are disposed to regard the reported successes as mere coincidences, and claim that the failures are seldom reported while the successes are widely heralded. The present writer presents the claims of this school to the attention of his readers, but without personally positively endorsing the idea. He is of the opinion that the data obtainable is not as yet sufficient to justify the strong claims made for the theory in some quarters; but, at the same time, he does not hesitate to say that there are many points of interest brought out in the presentation of the theory, and that many thoughtful persons seem to accept the same as reasonably well established and logical.

Another theory which has been heard of frequently of late years is that in which it is held that the ova are expelled in alternating sex, each month. Thus, if a male ovum is expelled in January, the February ovum will be a female one, according to this theory. Under this theory if the date of conception of a child be ascertained, and the sex of the child noted at its birth, it is a simple matter to count forward from the menstrual period following which the child was conceived, and thus determine whether the ovum of any succeeding period is male or female. It should be noted, however, that the periods are regulated by the lunar months, and not the calendar months. The fact that twins of different sexes are sometimes born would seem to disturb this theory—but not more than any other theory of sex-determination voluntarily produced, for that matter. The several schools explain this apparent discrepancy by the familiar saying that "exceptions prove the rule."

Another theory of sex-determination is that which holds that when conception occurs within a few days after the last day of menstruation, the child will be a girl; and that when conception occurs at a later period, the child will be a boy. Methods and systems based upon this theory are also reported as being reasonably successful in producing satisfactory results. But, inasmuch as there appears to be a great difference in individual women in this respect (even according to the claims of this school of sex-determination), it would seem that it would be difficult to proceed with certainty in the matter in most cases. One of the writers advocating this method, says: "Conception within five days after the end of the menstrual period is almost certain to produce a girl child; within five days to ten days, it may be either a boy or a girl; from ten to fifteen days, it is almost sure to be a boy; from eighteen to twenty-five days is the period of probable sterility, in which conception is extremely unlikely to occur."

In conclusion, it may be said that Nature undoubtedly has certain rules of sex-determination which govern in these cases; and that it is possible if not indeed probable that these rules may some day be discovered by man, and turned to account; but that it is very doubtful whether the secret has as yet been solved by the investigators. The writer may be pardoned for suggesting that, in his opinion, if the discovery is ever made it will likely be found to be very simple—so simple that we have probably overlooked it because it was in too plain sight to attract our attention. Nature's methods are usually very simple, when once discovered. She hides her processes from man by making them simple, it would seem.

LESSON X
WHAT BIRTH CONTROL IS, AND IS NOT

The student of the progress of human affairs, or even the average person whose knowledge of the doings of mankind is derived from a hasty and casual reading of the daily newspapers and the popular magazines, cannot plead ignorance of the growing interest in the general subject which is embraced within the content of the term "Birth Control."

But while the general meaning of the term is at least vaguely grasped by the average member of the human crowd—the individual to whom we refer as "the man on the street"—we find a startling condition of mental confusion and often positive misconception concerning the essence and spirit of the general idea expressed by the term in question.

While the fact is a reflection upon the average intelligence of the general public, it must be admitted that to the average person, or "the man on the street," Birth Control means simply the teaching and practice of certain methods whereby men and women may indulge their sexual appetites, in or out of marriage, without incurring the liability or risk of conception and child-bearing. The average person does not stop to consider that such teachings and practices do not constitute "Birth Control" at all, but are, rather, merely the theory and practice of Birth Prevention, desirable only to those who seek sexual indulgences without being called upon to shoulder the responsibilities attached by Nature to the physical sexual union of men and women.

The term "**control**" does not mean "prohibition," or "prevention"; but, on the contrary, means "governing, regulating, or managing influence." Birth Control, in the true meaning of the term, does not mean the prevention or prohibition of the birth of children, but rather the encouragement of the birth of children under the best possible conditions and the discouragement of the birth of children under improper or unfavorable conditions.

Birth Control, in the true meaning of the term, does not mean theories and practices which would tend to reduce the population of the civilized countries of the world, but rather theories and practice which would inevitably result in the production of an adequate ratio of increase in the population of such countries, not only by reason of a normal birth-rate, but also by reason of a diminishing death-rate among infants—by the production of healthier children, accompanied by the raising of the standard of the average child born in such countries.

Birth Control, in the true meaning of the term, therefore, is seen to consist not of the **prohibition** or **prevention** of human offspring, but rather of the **governing, regulating, and managing** of the production of human offspring, under the inspiration of the highest ideals and under the direction of the highest reason, for the purpose of the advancement and welfare of the race and that of the individuals composing the race. Instead of being an anti-social and anti-moral propaganda, Birth Control when rightly understood is perceived to be in accordance with the highest social aims and aspirations, and in accordance with the highest and purest morality of the race.

Much of the opposition toward the general movement of Birth Control which has been manifested by many well-meaning, though misinformed, persons, has arisen by reason of the erroneous conception and understanding of the term itself, and of misleading information concerning the true nature of the best teachings on the subject. This prejudice has been heightened by certain zealous but ill-balanced advocates of the general movement who have overemphasized the incidental feature of the limitation of offspring under certain conditions, and who have appealed to the attention and interest merely of those who wished to escape the responsibilities of parenthood. This has caused much sorrow and distress to the many persons who have the highest ideals and results in view, and who deplore this unbalanced propaganda under the name, and apparently under the cloak of the general movement. Such persons have felt inclined to cry aloud "Good Lord, deliver us from our so-called friends!"

One of the most distressing features of the popular prejudice against Birth Control, arising from a total misconception of the subject, has been the widely spread and popularly accepted notion that Birth Control is practically analogous to abortion—or, at the best, but a more refined and less repulsive and less dangerous form of abortion. In view of the fact that one of the important results sought to be obtained by a scientific knowledge of Birth Control actually is the prevention and avoidance of the crime of abortion which has wrought such terrible havoc among the women of civilized countries, it is most distressing and discouraging to the conscientious and high-minded advocates of Birth Control to have it said and believed that their teachings encourage and justify abortion.

A reference to any standard dictionary or textbook will reveal the fact that "Abortion" means: "the premature expulsion of the human embryo or foetus; miscarriage voluntarily induced or produced," etc. It is seen at a glance that the essence and meaning of abortion consists in the destruction of the human embryo which has resulted from conception. The embryo human child must already exist in its elemental form, before it can be destroyed by abortion. Therefore, if no such embryo form exists, it cannot be destroyed, and therefore there can be no abortion in such a case. And, it may positively be stated, no true advocate of Birth Control can possibly justify, much less advocate, the destruction of the human embryo or foetus, which act constitutes abortion. The difference between true Birth Control teachings and methods, and that of the advocates of abortion, is as great as the difference between the two poles. Instead of the two being identical or similar, they are diametrically opposed one to the other—they are logical "opposites," each the antithesis of the other.

Even in those forms or phases of the Birth Control propaganda in which the use of "contraceptives," or "preventatives" is considered justified in certain cases—and these forms and phases are far from being the most important, as all students of the subject know—even in these exceptional forms and phases of the general subject the idea of abortion is combatted, and never justified or encouraged. A "contraceptive" agency merely tends to prevent or obviate undesirable conception; it never acts to destroy the result of previous and accomplished conception. A "contraceptive" merely prevents the union of the male and female elements of reproduction, and consequently the process from which evolves the foetus or embryo. A leading medical authority has said regarding this distinction: "In inducing abortion, one destroys something already formed—a foetus or an embryo, a fertilized ovum, a potential human being. In prevention, however, one merely prevents chemically or mechanically the spermatozoa from coming in contact with the ovum. There is no greater sin or crime in this than there is in simple abstinence, in refraining from sexual intercourse."

What then must we say when we consider the higher and more advanced forms and phases of Birth Control, those phases and forms which may be said to be mental or emotional "contraceptives," rather than physical? Surely these cannot be considered as identical with or similar to abortion. And when we consider those phases and forms of Birth Control which are concerned with Pre-Natal Culture—the culture of the child before its birth —can one, even though he be intensely prejudiced against Birth Control, assert that there is to be found here anything which in any way whatsoever can be considered as relating to the theory or practice of abortion? And what must we say of the still higher phases in which the teachings are concerned with the mental and physical preparation of the parents prior to the conception of the child, to the end that the child may have the best possible physiological and psychological basis for its future well-being? Is not this the very antithesis and opposite of all that concerns abortion or abortive methods?

The trouble about all great movements designed for the benefit of the human race is that at the beginning there is attracted to the movement, by reason of its novelty and "newness," certain elements which seize upon certain incidental features of the general idea, make them their own while excluding or ignoring the more important things, and then exploit these incidental features in a sensational way, thereby attracting public attention and gaining much undesirable notoriety, and as a consequence bringing discredit and disfavor, prejudice and misunderstanding, to the general movement.

Birth Control has passed through this apparently inevitable experience, and has suffered greatly thereby. But the Light is being thrown on the Dark Places, and the more intelligent portion of the public is beginning to realize that there is another side to the shield of Birth Control. And, as a consequence, much of the original prejudice is disappearing, and a new understanding of the subject is arising in the minds of many of the best individuals of the race. It is the purpose of this book to help to dispel the ignorance and misconception concerning this great subject of Birth Control, and to aid in presenting the higher and nobler aspects of the general movement to the attention of those who are concerned with the advance and progress of the race as a whole, and of the individual members thereof.

The student of the subject of Birth Control will fall into grievous error if he begins his consideration of the subject under the impression that the questions concerned therein are new to the world of living things. If the process of Birth Control were something which had suddenly sprung into existence in the consciousness of man, without having an antecedent activity in the history of the race, and of living creatures in general, we might well hesitate to go further in the matter without the most serious and prolonged consideration of the entire principle by the careful thought of the wisest of the race. But while such consideration is advisable, as in the case of any and all important problems presenting themselves for solution and judgment, it is found that those so considering the subject have a sound and firm foundation upon which to base their thought and to test their conclusions.

As many thoughtful students of the subject have pointed out to us, the question of Birth Control has been with the race practically since the beginning of human history; and it has its correspondences in the instinctive actions of the lower forms of life. The chief difference is that we are now seeking to deal with these problems consciously, voluntarily, and deliberately, whereas in the past the race has dealt with them more or less unconsciously, by methods of trial and error, through perpetual experiment which has often proved costly but which has all the more clearly brought out the real course of natural processes.

We cannot hope to solve problems so ancient and so deeply rooted as these by merely the rational methods of yesterday and today. To be of value our rational methods must be the revelation in deliberate consciousness of unconscious methods which go far back into the remote past. Our deliberate methods will not be sound except in so far as they are a continuation of those methods which, in the slow evolution of life, have been found sound and progressive on the plane of instinct. This is particularly true in the case of those among us who desire their own line of conduct in the matter to be so closely in accord with natural law, or the law of creation, that to question it would be impious.

It may be accepted without an extended argument or presentation of evidence that at the outset the prime object of Nature seems to have been that of Reproduction. There is evident, without doubt, an effort on the part of Nature to secure economy of method in the attainment of ever greater perfection in the process of reproduction, but we cannot deny that the primary motive seems to be that of reproduction pure and simple. The tendency toward reproduction is indeed so fundamental in Nature that it is impressed with the greatest emphasis upon every living thing. And, as careful thinkers have told us "the course of evolution seems to have been more of an effort to slow down reproduction than to furnish it with new facilities."

Reproduction appears in the history of life even before sex manifests itself. The lower forms of animal and plant life oftener produce themselves without the aid of sex, and some authorities have argued that the presence of sex differentiation serves rather to check active propagation rather than to increase it. If quantity, without regard to quality or variation, be the object of Nature, then that purpose would have been better served by withholding sex-differentiation than by evolving it. As Professor Coulter, a leading American botanist, has well said: "The impression one gains of sexuality is that it represents reproduction under peculiar difficulties."

To those who find it difficult to assimilate this somewhat startling idea, we now present a brief statement of the infinitely greater facility toward reproduction manifested by living creatures lacking in sex-differentiation as compared with those possessing it. It is seen that bacteria among primitive plants, and protozoa among primitive animals, are patterns of very rapid and prolific reproduction, though sex begins to appear in a rudimentary form in very lowly forms of life. A single infusorian becomes in a week the ancestor of millions, that is to say, of far more individuals than could proceed under the most favorable conditions from a pair of elephants in five centuries; and Huxley has calculated that the progeny of a single parthenogenetic aphis, under favorable circumstances, would in a few months outweigh the whole population of China. It must be noted, however, that this proviso "under favorable circumstances" reveals the weak point of Nature's early method of reproduction by enormously rapid multiplication. Creatures so easily produced are easily destroyed; and Nature, apparently in consequence, wastes no time in imparting to them the qualities needed for a high form of life and living.

And, even after sex differentiation had attained a considerable degree of development, Nature seemed slow to abandon her original plan of rapid multiplication of individuals. Among insects so far advanced as the white ants, the queen lays eggs at the enormous rate of 80,000 a day during her period of active life. Higher in the scale, we find the female herring laying 70,000 eggs at one period of delivery. But in both of these cases we find the manifestation of that apparently invariable rule of Nature, viz., that **a high birth-rate is accompanied by a heavy death-rate**, whether that high death-rate be caused by natural enemies, wars, or disease.

At a certain stage of the evolutionary process, Nature seems to have awakened to a realization of the fact that it was better, from every point of view, to produce **a few** superior beings rather than a vast number of inferior ones. Here, at last, Nature discloses a heretofore hidden aim, namely, the production of quality rather than quantity; and once she has started on this new path, she has pursued it with even greater eagerness than that of reproduction pure and simple. And here we pause to note a principle laid down by the students of Evolution, viz., that **advancing evolution is accompanied by declining fertility**.

This new stage of Nature's processes is marked by a constant and invariable manifestation of diminished number of offspring, accompanied by an increased amount of time and care in the creation and breeding of each of the young creatures. Accompanying this, we find that the reproductive life of the creature is shortened, and confined to more or less special periods; these periods beginning much later, and ending much earlier, and even during their continuance tending to operate in cycles of activity. Here, we see, **Nature, grown wiser by experience, herself began to exercise her power in the direction of Birth Control—the use of preventive checks on reproduction**.

A writer has said along these lines: "As reproduction slackened, evolution was greatly accelerated. A highly important and essential aspect of this greater individuation is a higher survival value. The more complex and better equipped creature can meet and subdue difficulties and dangers to which the more lowly organized creature that came before—produced wholesale in a way which Nature seems to look back on as cheap and nasty —succumbed helplessly without an effort. The idea of economy began to assert itself in the world. It became clear in the course of evolution that it is better to produce really good and highly efficient organisms, at whatever cost, than to be content with cheap production on a wholesale scale. They allowed greater developmental progress to be made, and they lasted better. Even before man began it was proved in the animal world that **the death-rate falls as the birth-rate falls**."

Let us compare the lowly herring with the highly evolved elephant. The herring multiplies with enormous rapidity and on a vast scale, and it possesses a very small brain, and is almost totally unequipped to grapple with the special difficulties of its life, to which it succumbs on a wholesale scale. A single elephant is carried for about two years in its mother's womb, and is carefully guarded by her for many years after birth; it possesses a large brain, and its muscular system is as remarkable for its delicacy as for its power, and is guided by the most sensitive perceptions. It is fully equipped for all the dangers of life, save for those which have been introduced by the subtle ingenuity of modern man. Though a single pair of elephants produces so few offspring, yet their high cost is justified, for each of them has a reasonable chance of surviving to old age. This contrast, from the point of view of reproduction, of the herring and the elephant, well illustrates the principle of evolution previously referred to. It brings clearly into view the difference between Nature's earlier and her later methods— the ever increasing preference for quality over quantity. Unless we grasp this underlying principle of Nature in its wider aspects we may fail to perceive its operations in the case of man, which latter we may now consider.

It is, of course, impossible to speak positively regarding the birth-rate and death-rate of the pre-historic primitive races of mankind, for there is not data upon which to base such a report. But reasoning upon the basis of conditions existing among the primitive tribes of the present time we are justified in holding that in the early stages of the evolution of the race there was manifested a high birth-rate and a correspondingly high death-rate. Upon the basis of conditions now existing among savage tribes it would appear that primitive man has a higher birth-rate than the average of mankind today, and likewise a higher death-rate. The rapidly increasing number of children born to the tribe was counteracted by deaths among children caused by neglect, poverty, and disease. In some cases the population was prevented from becoming larger than the means of subsistence justified by the practice of infanticide.

As to the condition of the race in the early stages of "modern" civilization, we have modern Russia as a surviving instance of this stage. In modern Russia we find, side by side with the progress in neighboring nations, conditions which a few centuries ago existed all over Europe. Here we have an enormous birth-rate, and a terrible death-rate caused by ignorance, superstition, insanitation, filth, bad food, impure water, plagues, famines, and other accompaniments of overcrowding and misery. We find a mortality among young children which sometimes destroys more than half of the children born before they have attained the age of five years. As high as is the Russian birth-rate, it is a matter of record that at times the death-rate has actually exceeded it. And among the survivors there is found a startlingly large percentage of chronic and incurable diseases, with a large number of cases of blindness and other defects.

Similar results follow in China, where the birth-rate is exceptionally high, and the death-rate correspondingly large; and where there is a large percentage of inferior physical development and pathological defects, the evil conditions which produce death also tending to produce deterioration in the survivors. In both of these countries we have an example of the result of unrestricted reproduction, and unrestricted destruction—as among herrings, so among men. And yet this condition of unrestricted reproduction is the logical goal of certain persons who, inspired by the best possible intentions, in their ignorance and criminal rashness would dare to arrest that fall in the birth-rate which is now beginning to spread its influence in every civilized land.

In Western Europe before the nineteenth century the population increased very slowly. The enormous birth-rate was nearly equalled by the exceedingly heavy death-rate caused by plagues, pestilences, and famine, and by the frequent wars large and small. The mortality among young children was particularly heavy. Writers have pointed out that the old family records show frequently two or three children of the same Christian name, the first child having died and its name given to a successor.

During the last quarter of the eighteenth century, when machinery was introduced and a new industrial era opened, the birth-rate rose rapidly. Factories springing up gave increased support to many, and as children were employed as "hands" in the mills at an early age, the richest family was the one with most children. The population began to increase rapidly. But soon disease, misery, and poverty arose from filth and insanitation, immorality and crime, overcrowding and child-labor, drink and lack of sane courses of conduct.

In time, however, progress set in, and social reformers began the great movement for the betterment of the environment, sanitation, shorter hours of labor, and restriction of child-labor, factory regulation, etc. And when the environment is bettered, the death-rate drops, and the birth-rate accompanies it on its downward progress. As Leroy-Beaulieu says: "The first degree of prosperity in a rude population with few needs tends toward prolificness of reproduction; a later degree of prosperity, accompanied by all the feelings and ideas stimulated by the reduction of such prolificness."

The law of the reduction of reproduction in response to the improvement of environment is a natural law, arising from fixed biological principles. This is because when we improve the environment we improve the individual situated in that environment; and the improvement of the individual has always resulted in a check upon reproduction. We must remember, however, that this change is not the result of conscious or voluntary action; instead it is the result of unconscious activities and instinctive urge. As Sir Shirley Murphy has said: "Birth Control is a natural process, and though in civilized men, endowed with high intelligence, it necessarily works in some measure voluntarily and deliberately, it is probable that it also works, as in the evolution of the lower animals, to some extent automatically."

Science shows us that even among the most primitive micro-organisms; when placed under unfavorable conditions as to food and environment, they tend to pass into a reproductive phase and by sporulation or otherwise begin to produce new individuals rapidly. This, of course, because of the fact that their death-rate is increased, and an increased birth-rate must be manifested in order to maintain a balance. If the environment be improved, the death-rate decreases, and this is followed by a fall in the birth-rate, according to the constant laws of Nature manifesting in such cases.

The same law is seen to be manifested in the case of Man. Improve his environment, and his death-rate drops, which is accompanied by a falling birth-rate. Here, once more we see the application of the scientific axiom "Improve the environment and reproduction is checked." As Leroy-Beaulieu has said: "The tendency of civilization is to reduce the birth-rate." And as Professor Benjamin Moore has said: "Decreased reproduction is the simple biological reply to good economic conditions." And as Havelock Ellis has said: "Those who desire a higher birth-rate are desiring, whether they know it or not, the increase of poverty, ignorance, and wretchedness."

Among men, Birth Control has now evolved from the unconscious and instinctive phase, and is now unfolding and manifesting on the plane of conscious and voluntary activity. The influence of deliberate intention and conscious design is now one of the important factors in the process. Here at this point we reach a totally new aspect of reproduction. In the past stages of evolution the original impetus toward reproduction has been checked and directed by Nature, working along instinctive and unconscious lines; and the result has been an extreme diminution of the number of off-spring; a prolongation of the time devoted to the breeding and care of each new member of the family, in harmony with its greatly prolonged life; a spacing out of the intervals between the offspring; and, as a result, a vastly greater development of each individual, and an ever better equipment for the task of living. All this was slowly attained automatically, without any conscious volition on the part of the individuals, even when they were human beings, who were the agents.

Now, however, we are confronted with a change which we may regard as, in some respects, the most momentous sudden advance in the whole history of reproduction, namely, the process of reproductive progress now become conscious and deliberately volitional. Birth control, no longer automatic, is now being directed by human mind and will precisely to the attainment of ends which Nature has been struggling after for millions of years; and, being consciously and deliberately directed, it is now enabled to avoid many of the pitfalls into which the unconscious method fell.

Havelock Ellis says: "The control and limitation of reproductive activity by conscious and volitional effort is an attempt by open-eyed intelligence and foresight to attain those ends which Nature through untold generations has been painfully yet tirelessly struggling for. The deliberate co-operation of Man in the natural task of Birth Control represents an identification of the human will with what we may, if we choose, regard as the divinely appointed law of the world. We can well believe that the great pioneers, who, a century ago, acted in the spirit of this faith may have echoed the thought of Kepler when, on discovering his great planetary law, he exclaimed in rapture: 'O God! I think Thy thoughts after Thee!'"

The following brief general history of the modern Birth Control movement is quoted from Havelock Ellis, and will be of interest to students of the subject: "The pioneers of modern Birth Control were English. Among them Malthus occupies the first place. That distinguished man, in his great and influential work, 'The Principles of Population,' in 1798, emphasized the immense importance of foresight and self-control in procreation, and the profound significance of birth limitation for human welfare. Malthus, however, relied on ascetic self-restraint, a method which could only appeal to the few; he had nothing to say for the regulation of conception in intercourse. That was suggested twenty years later, very cautiously by James Mill, the father of John Stuart Mill, in the 'Encyclopaedia Britannica.' Four years afterwards, Mill's friend, the Radical reformer, Francis Place, advocated this method more clearly. Finally, in 1831, Robert Dale Owen, the son of the great Robert Owen, published his 'Moral Physiology,' in which he set forth the ways of preventing conception; while a little later the Drysdale brothers, ardent and unwearying philanthropists, devoted their energies to a propaganda which has been spreading ever since and has now conquered the whole civilized world.

"It was not, however, in England but in France, so often at the head of an advance in civilization, that Birth Control first firmly became established, and that the extravagantly high birth rate of earlier times began to fall; this happened in the first half of the nineteenth century, whether or not it was mainly due to voluntary control. In England the movement came later, and the steady decline in the English birth-rate, which is still proceeding, began in 1877. In the previous year there had been a famous prosecution of Bradlaugh and Mrs. Besant for disseminating pamphlets describing the methods of preventing conception; the charge was described by the Lord Chief Justice, who tried the case, as one of the most ill-advised and injudicious ever made in a court of justice. But it served an undesigned end by giving enormous publicity to the subject and advertising the methods it sought to suppress. There can be no doubt, however, that even apart from this trial the movement would have proceeded on the same lines. The times were ripe, the great industrial expansion had passed its first feverish phase, social conditions were improving, education was spreading. The inevitable character of the movement is indicated by the fact that at the very same time it began to be manifested all over Europe, indeed in every civilized country of the world.

"At the present time the birth-rate (as well as usually the death-rate) is falling in every country of the world sufficiently civilized to possess statistics of its own vital movement. The fall varies in rapidity. It has been considerable in the more progressive countries; it has lingered in the more backward countries. If we examine the latest statistics for Europe, we find that every country, without exception, with a progressive and educated population, and a fairly high state of social well-being, presents a birth-rate below 30 per 1,000. We also find that every country in Europe in which the mass of the people are primitive, ignorant, or in a socially unsatisfactory condition (even although the governing classes may be progressive or ambitious) shows a birth-rate of above 30 per 1,000. France, Great Britain, Belgium, Holland, the Scandinavian countries, and Switzerland are in the first group. Russia, Austro-Hungary, Italy, Spain, and the Balkan countries are in the second group. The German Empire was formerly in the second group, but now comes within the first group, and has carried on the movement so energetically that the birth-rate of Berlin is already below that of London, and that at the present rate of decline the birth-rate of the German Empire will before long sink to that of France. Outside Europe, in the United States just as much as in Australia and New Zealand, the same progressive movement is proceeding with equal activity."

The same authority sums up the present attitude of the advocates of scientific and rational Birth Control, as follows: "The wide survey of the question of birth limitation has settled the question of the desirability of the adoption of preventing conception, and finally settled those who would waste out time with their fears that it is not right to control conception. We know now on whose side are the laws of God and Nature. We realize that in exercising control over the entrance gate of life we are not fully performing, consciously and deliberately, a great human duty, but carrying on rationally a beneficial process which has, more blindly and wastefully, been carried on since the beginning of the world. There are still a few persons ignorant enough or foolish enough to fight against the advance of civilization in this matter; we can well afford to leave them severely alone, knowing that in a few years all of them will have passed away. It is not our business to defend the control of birth, but simply discuss how we may most wisely exercise that control."

LESSON XI
THE FETICH OF THE BIRTH-RATE

To the student of the progress of the human race the consideration of the state of public opinion regarding the Birth-rate of nations is of great interest. To the careful observer there is evident the gradual evolution of intelligent public opinion on this subject even in the comparatively short space of time in which the present generation has played its part on the great stage of human development.

Public opinion on this subject during the period named may be said to have passed through three general stages. These stages are, of course, more clearly defined among the peoples of the most prosperous and intelligent countries, as for instance, in Western Europe and America, and particularly in England, France, and the United States. While the peoples of certain of these countries have passed through these stages somewhat more rapidly than have others, still it is perceived that each of these peoples have in the main followed the same general course.

The first stage of this evolution of popular opinion may be said to have been begun about 1850, and to have ended about 1880. In this stage the ideal of a large and rapidly increasing birth-rate became a popular fetich before which all men and women were supposed to fall down and render worship. In this period public opinion manifested great satisfaction and joy in the evidences of a high and rapidly increasing birth-rate. It was held that this increasing birth-rate tended toward the success and glory of the particular nation, and incidentally to the race as a whole. The idea of **Quantity** was elevated to the throne of public favor, and the question of **Quality** was ignored or overlooked.

This period was one of an unusual expansion of industry, and the rising birth-rate was regarded as a token that the world was destined to be exploited and eventually governed by the people of those nations who were able to demonstrate the greatest efficiency in industrial pursuits, and who at the same time were wise enough to increase their respective populations by an increasing birth-rate. The populace were excited by the idea of the dominance and prosperity of their own countrymen, while the leaders of industry were delighted with the idea of an increasing supply of laborers which would tend to keep down the rate of wages which otherwise would have reached proportions which would have interfered with competition with other countries. At the same time, the militarists were secretly delighted by the signs of an increasing supply of military material with which to build up gigantic armies.

A writer on the state of public opinion on this subject during this period has well said: "It seemed to the more exuberant spirits that a vast British Empire, or a mighty Pan-German, might be expected to cover the whole world. France, with its low and falling birth-rate, was looked down at with a contempt as a decadent country inhabited with a degenerate population. No attempt to analyze the birth-rate, to ascertain what are really the biological, social, and economic accompaniments of a high birth-rate, made any impression on the popular mind. They were drowned in a general shout of exultation."

But this period of uncritical optimism was followed by a natural reaction. The pendulum stopped in its course, and soon began to swing in the opposite direction. Here, about 1880, the second stage may be said to have begun. Public opinion began to manifest a subtle change, and this mental attitude was accompanied by a physical manifestation in the form of a decreasing birth-rate. The rate of births began to fall rapidly, and has continued to fall steadily since that time.

The writer above quoted from says of this second period: "In France the birth-rate fell slowly, in Italy more rapidly, and in England and Prussia still more rapidly. As, however, the fall began earliest in France, the birth-rate was lower there than in the other countries named. For the same reason it was lower in England than in Prussia, although England stands in this respect at almost exactly the same distance from Prussia today (1917) as thirty years ago, the fall having occurred at the same rate in both countries. It is quite possible that in the future it may become more rapid in Prussia than in England, for the birth-rate of Berlin is lower than the birth-rate of London, and urbanization is proceeding at a more rapid rate in Germany than in England."

It is not difficult to arrive at the psychological reason underlying this great change in public opinion, as manifested in this second stage. In the first place, the wonderful era of world-expansion was arrested, by natural causes well understood by students of sociology. The ambitious dreams of world-empires were rudely interrupted. Moreover, public opinion was being affected by a quiet education along the lines of sociology and economics.

The working classes began to perceive, on the one hand, the tendency of overpopulation to hold down, or even decrease, the scale of wages. The evils of over-production, and of under-consumption were dimly perceived. And, on the other hand, the capitalists began to perceive that another factor was at work—one which they had failed to include in their optimistic calculations. Instead of the cheaper wage rate which they had expected by reason of the over-abundance of human material, they found that the growth of popular education in the democratic countries had caused the working classes to demand greater comforts of life, and to oppose the cheapening of human labor. And at the same time, the masses began to revolt against the idea of raising children to become "cannon fodder" for ambitious autocratic rulers. The masses began to protest against selling their labor and their lives so cheaply.

These changed viewpoints of the working classes began to result in attempts on their part to form associations to resist the tendency on the part of capitalists to force down the scale of wages to fit the increased population. Trade unions flourished and became powerful, and the same impulse carried many into the ranks of socialism, and still beyond into the fold of anarchism and syndicalism. And, here note this significant fact, with these new perceptions and these new movements among the masses, **the birth-rate began to fall rapidly**.

The writer above quoted from says of this period: "The pessimists were faced by horrors on both sides. On the one hand, they saw that the ever-increasing rate of human production which seemed to them the essential condition of national, social, even moral progress, had not only stopped but was steadily diminishing. On the other hand, they saw that, even so far as it was maintained, it involved, under modern conditions, nothing but social commotion and economic disturbance. There are still many pessimists of this class alive among us even today, alike in England and Germany, but a new generation is growing up, and this question is now entering another phase."

It would seem that the race is now well started in the third period, phase, or stage of this conception of the birth-rate. Even the Great War is not likely to seriously interrupt its ultimate progress, though conditions in all civilized countries will unquestionably be disturbed by the unusual conditions now prevailing and caused by the great conflict. The spirit of this third stage seems to be that the Truth is to be found between the two extremes, viz.: (1) the extreme of passive optimism of the first stage; and (2) the extreme of passive pessimism of the second stage. It realizes that there is excellent ground for hope in better things; but it equally realizes that hope alone is vain, and will accomplish nothing unless it is accompanied with and directed by a clear intellectual vision manifested in individual and social action based on that clear intellectual vision.

The writer above quoted from says of this developing period: "It is today beginning to be seen that the old notion of progress by means of reckless multiplication is vain. It can only be effected at a ruinous cost of death, disease, poverty, and misery. We see this in the past history of Western Europe, as we still see it in the history of Russia. Any progress effected along that line—if 'progress' it can be called—is now barred, for it is utterly opposed to those democratic conceptions which are ever gaining greater influence among us. Moreover, we are now better able to analyze demographic phenomena, and are no longer satisfied with any crude statements regarding the birth-rate. We realize that they need interpretation. They have to be considered in relation to the sex-constitution and the age-constitution of the population, and **above all, they must be viewed in relation to the infant mortality rate**.

"The bad aspect of the French birth-rate is not so much its lowness as that it is accompanied by a high infantile mortality. The fact that the German birth-rate is higher than the English ceases to be a matter of satisfaction when it is realized that German infantile mortality is vastly greater than English. **A high birth-rate is no sign of a high civilization. But we are beginning to feel that a high infantile death-rate is a sign of a very inferior civilization. A low birth-rate with a low infant death-rate not only produces the same increase in population as a high birth-rate with**

a high death-rate, which always accompanies it (for there are no examples of a high birth-rate with a low death-rate), but it produces it in a way which is far more worthy of our admiration in this matter than the way of Russia and China where opposite conditions prevail."

The evolutionary process which all students of sociology clearly perceive to have been underway in the matter of the attitude of public opinion toward the birth-rate, and which is now underway with increased impetus, is perceived to be a natural process. It is a natural process which has been underway from the beginning of the living world. For a long time it operated and manifested along unconscious and instinctive lines of activity, but now it has emerged into the light of human consciousness and manifests along the lines of conscious, voluntary, and deliberate human action.

In its present state of evolutionary progress human thought along these lines has found expression in what is generally known as "Birth Control." The process which has been working slowly through the ages, attaining every new forward step with waste and pain, is henceforth destined to be carried out voluntarily, in the light of human reason, foresight, and self-restraint. The rise of Birth Control may be said to correspond with the rise of social and sanitary science in the first half of the nineteenth century, and to be indeed an essential part of that movement.

The new doctrine of Birth Control is now firmly established in all the most progressive and enlightened countries of Europe, notably in France and England; in Germany, where formerly the birth-rate was very high, Birth Control has developed with extraordinary rapidity during the present century. In Holland its principles and practice are freely taught by physicians and nurses to the mothers of the people, with the result that there is in Holland no longer any necessity for unwanted babies, and this small country possesses the proud privilege of the lowest death-rate in Europe.

In the free and enlightened Democratic communities on the other side of the globe, in Australia and New Zealand, the same principles and practice are generally accepted, with the same beneficent results. On the other hand, in the more backward and ignorant countries of Europe, Birth Control is still little known, and death and disease flourish. This is the case in those eight European countries which come at the bottom of the list of the Birth

Control scale, and in which the birth-rate is the highest and the death-rate the heaviest—the two rates maintaining such a constant correspondence as to lead to the inevitable conclusion that they are associated as cause and effect.

But even in the more progressive countries Birth Control has not been established without a struggle, which has frequently ended in a hypocritical compromise, its principles being publicly ignored or denied and its practice privately accepted. For, at the great and vitally important point in human progress which Birth-Control represents, we see really the conflict of two moralities. The morality of the ancient world is here confronted by the morality of the new world.

The old morality, knowing nothing of science and the process of Nature as worked out in the evolution of life, contented itself with assuming as a basis the early chapters of Genesis in which the children of Noah are represented as entering an empty earth which it is their business to populate diligently. So it came about that for this morality, still innocent of eugenics, recklessness was almost a virtue. Children were held to be given by God; if they died or were afflicted by congenital disease, it was the dispensation of God, and, whatever imprudence the parents might commit, the pathetic faith still ruled that "God will provide."

But in the new morality it is realized that in these matters Divine action can only be made manifest in human action, that is to say through the operation of our own enlightened reason and resolved will. Prudence, foresight, self-restraint—virtues which old morality looked down upon with benevolent contempt—assume a position of first importance. In the eyes of the new morality the ideal woman is no longer the meek drudge condemned to endless and often ineffectual child-bearing, but the free and instructed woman, able to look before and after, trained in a sense of responsibility alike to herself and to the race, and determined to have no children but the best.

Such were the two moralities which came into conflict during the nineteenth century. They are irreconcilable and each firmly rooted, one in ancient religion and tradition, the other in progressive science and reason. Nothing was possible in such a clash of opposing ideas but a feeble and confused compromise such as we find still prevailing in various countries of Old Europe. This is not a satisfactory solution, however inevitable, and is especially unsatisfactory by the consequent obscurantism which placed difficulties in the way of spreading a knowledge of the methods of Birth Control among the masses of the population. For the result has been that while the more enlightened and educated have exercised a control over the size of their families, the poorer and more ignorant—those who should have been offered every facility and encouragement to follow in the same path—have been left, through a conspiracy of silence, to carry on helplessly the bad customs of their forefathers. This social neglect has had the result that the superior family stocks have been tampered by the recklessness of the inferior stocks.

In America, we find the two moralities in active conflict today. Until recently America has meekly accepted at the hand of Old Europe the traditional prescription. On the surface, the ancient morality had been complacently, almost unquestionably, accepted in America, even to the extent of tacitly permitting the existence of a vast extension of abortion, under the surface of society— a criminal practice which ever flourishes where Birth Control is neglected.

But today, a new movement is perceptible in America. It would seem that, almost in a flash, America has awakened to the true significance of the issue. With that direct vision of hers, that swift practicality of action, and above all, that sense of the democratic nature of all social progress, we see her resolutely beginning to face this great problem. In her vigorous tongue she is demanding "What is all this secrecy about, anyway? Let us turn on the Light!" And the best authorities agree that America's answer to the demand will be of the greatest importance, and of immense significance to the whole world.

In concluding this portion of our discussion, I ask my readers to consider the following quotations from writers who have touched upon the question of the stimulation of the birth-rate by the State, for the purpose of military policy. These quotations speak for themselves, and need but little comment.

The first authority, a German, whose name has escaped me for the moment, laments the falling birth-rate in his country, and urges his own nation to stimulate it by offering bounties; he says: "Woe to us if we follow the example of the wicked and degenerate people of other nations. Our nation needs men. We have to populate the earth, and to carry the blessings of our Kultur all over the world. In executing that high mission we cannot have too much human material in defending ourselves against the aggression of other nations who are jealous of us and our achievements and progress. Let us promote parentage by law; let us repress by law every influence which may encourage a falling birth-rate; otherwise there is nothing left us but speedy national disaster, complete and irremediable."

Havelock Ellis, an Englishman, says: "In Germany for years past it has been difficult to take up a serious periodical without finding some anxiously statistical article about the falling birth-rate, and some wild recommendations for its arrest. For it is the militaristic German who of all Europeans is most worried by this fall; indeed Germans often even refuse to recognize it. Thus today we find Professor Gruber declaring that if the population of the German Empire continues to grow at the rate of the first five years of the present century, it will have reached 250,000,000 at the end of the century. By such a vast increase in population, the Professor complacently concludes, 'Germany will be rendered invulnerable.' But Gruber's estimate is entirely fallacious. German births have fallen, roughly speaking, about 1 per 1,000 of the population, every year since the beginning of the century, and it would be equally reasonable to estimate that if they continue to fall at the present rate (which we cannot, of course, anticipate) births will altogether have ceased in Germany before the end of the century. The German birth-rate reached its climax forty years ago (1871-1880) with 40.7 per 1,000; in 1906 it was 34 per 1,000; in 1909 it was 31 per 1,000; in 1912 it was 28 per 1,000; in an almost measurable period of time, in all probability before the end of the century, it will have reached the same low level as that of France, when there will be but little difference between the 'invulnerability' of France and of Germany, a consummation which, for the world's sake, is far more devoutly to be wished than that anticipated by Gruber."

Writers of Teutonic sympathies have asserted that the aggressive attitude of Germany at the beginning of the Great War was to be legitimately explained and apologized for on the ground that the War was the inevitable expansive outcome of the abnormally high birth-rate of Germany in recent times. Dr. Dernburg, the German statesman, said not very long ago: "The expansion of the German nation has been so extraordinary during the past twenty-five years that the conditions existing before the war had become insupportable." Another writer has said: "Of later years there has arisen a movement among German women for bringing abortion into honor and repute, so that it may be carried out openly and with the aid of the best physicians. This movement has been supported by lawyers and social reformers of high position."

Thus, it would seem that a birth-rate stimulated by unusual circumstances or by deliberate State encouragement, seemingly draws upon it the operation of natural laws which tend to increase its death-rate by War, as well as by an increased number of abortions, and an increased death-rate. It would seem as natural laws operate to bring down the population to normal by war if the other factors do not operate sufficiently rapidly and efficiently.

Havelock Ellis makes the following interesting statement: "If we survey the belligerent nations in the war we may say that those who took the initiative in drawing it on, or at all events were most prepared to welcome it, were Germany, Austria, Serbia, and Russia—all nations with a high birth-rate, and in which the fall of the birth-rate has not yet had time to permeate. On the other hand, of the belligerent peoples of today, all indications point to the French as the people most intolerant, silently but deeply, of the war they are so ably and heroically waging. Yet the France of the present, with the lowest birth-rate, was a century ago the France of a birth-rate higher than that of Germany today, and at that time the most militarist and aggressive of nations, a perpetual menace to Europe."

Finally, let us quote Havelock Ellis once more; he says: "When we realize these facts we are also enabled to realize how futile, how misplaced and how mischievous it is to raise the cry of 'Race Suicide.' It is futile because no outcry can affect a world-wide movement of civilization. It is misplaced because the rise and fall of the population is not a matter of birth-rate alone, but of the birth-rate combined with the death-rate, and while we cannot expect to touch the former we can influence the latter. It is mischievous because by fighting against a tendency which is not only inevitable but altogether beneficial, we blind ourselves to the advance of civilization and risk the misdirection of our energies. How far this blindness may be carried we see in the false patriotism of those who in the decline of the birth-rate, fancy they see the ruin of their own particular country, oblivious of the fact that we are concerned with a phenomenon of world-wide extension. The whole tendency of civilization is to reduce the birth-rate. We may go further, and assert with the distinguished German economist, Roscher, that the chief cause of the superiority of a highly civilized state over lower stages of civilization is precisely a greater degree of forethought and self-control in marriage and child-bearing. Instead of talking about Race Suicide, we should do well to observe at what an appalling rate, even yet, the population is increasing; and we should note that it is everywhere the poorest and most primitive countries, and in every country (as in Germany) the poorest regions, which show the highest birth-rate."

The same authority says: "One last resort the would-be patriotic alarmist seeks when all others fail. He is good enough to admit that a general decline in the birth-rate might be beneficial. But, he points out, it affects social classes unequally. It is initiated, not by the degenerate and unfit, with whom we could well dispense, but by the very best classes in the community, the well-to-do and the educated. One is inclined to remark, at once, that a social change initiated by its best social class is scarcely likely to be pernicious. Where, it may be asked, if not among the most educated classes, is any process of amelioration to be initiated? We cannot make the world topsy-turvy to suit the convenience of topsy-turvy minds. All social movements tend to begin at the top and to permeate downwards. This has been the case with the decline of the birth-rate, but it is already well marked among the working classes, and has only failed to touch the lowest stratum of all, too weak-minded and too reckless to be amenable to ordinary social motives. The rational method of meeting this situation is not a propaganda in favor of procreation—a truly imbecile propaganda, since it is only carried out and only likely to be carried out, by the very class which we wish to sterilize—but rather by a wise policy of regulative eugenics. We have to create the motives, and it is not an impossible task, which will act even upon the weak-minded and reckless lowest social stratum."

LESSON XII
THE ARGUMENT FOR BIRTH CONTROL

Let us now consider the general and special arguments advanced in favor of rational and scientific Birth Control, as stated by the advocates thereof.

General Argument. The general argument in favor of Birth Control may well be begun by the statement that rational and scientific Birth Control is not the fixing upon the race of a new and unfamiliar practice or policy, but is rather the scientific correction of a practice and policy which is now followed by the majority of married persons in civilized countries, though in a bungling, unscientific, and frequently a harmful manner. The modern advocates of scientific methods of Birth Control seek to replace these bungling, unscientific, and frequently harmful methods by sane, scientific, harmless methods, approved of by capable physicians and other experienced and capable authorities, and under the sanction of the law rather than contrary to it.

The advocates of Birth Control seek to place upon a scientific basis, under cover and protection of the law, a subject which heretofore has been but imperfectly known, and more imperfectly practiced in some form by the majority of married couples, and which has heretofore been under condemnation of the law so far as concerned the actual dissemination of information concerning methods of contraception. They hold that it is the veriest hypocrisy to pretend ignorance of the fact that the great majority of married couples in civilized communities know and practice to some extent contraceptive methods—usually imperfectly and bunglingly, it must be added.

One has but to consider the families of married couples, and to count their children, to become aware that at least some form of contraception has been known and practiced in many cases. This is particularly true of the more intelligent and cultured members of civilized society, among whom we find large families of children to be the exception, and small families to be the general rule. Among the less intelligent and uncultured classes the reverse of this condition is found.

It is hypocritical folly to assert that these small families to be found among the more intelligent classes of society are due to the fact that the husbands and wives are physically incapable of procreating off-spring—the mere suggestion produces an incredulous smile from the reader. No one who is acquainted with the habits and customs of married people would in good faith offer such an explanation. Rather is it tacitly acknowledged by all thinking persons that such married couples practice some form of Birth Control, or else commit the crime of abortion. All physicians, particularly those who practice in the large cities, are fully informed as to the appalling facts concerning the prevalence of abortion among the women of the "respectable" classes, and are likewise fully informed as to the terrible consequences so frequently arising from this criminal course.

The question, then, to many intelligent persons is not so much that of "Should contraception be employed in order to avoid excessively large families?" as that of "Should not contraception be employed to obviate the crime of abortion with its terrible train of consequences?" And the Birth Control propaganda which is so vigorously underway in all civilized countries may be stated to be designed for the following purposes: (1) to replace abortion, and other harmful methods of restricting the size of families, with rational and scientific methods of contraception; and (2) to supply to married persons the best scientific knowledge concerning the regulation of the size of families, and the methods of producing the best kind of children, under the best conditions, and at the times best adapted for their proper care and well-being. These advocates of the Betterment of the Race face the facts of human nature and married life fearlessly, instead of trying to cover them over with pretty words and sentimental generalities. They take "things as they are," and not as certain persons insist that "they should be"—they live in a world of facts and try to better things as they find them, instead of trying to live in a fool's paradise and contenting themselves with denying the existence of the facts which they consider "ugly."

Dr. William J. Robinson, one of the leading American workers in the field of Birth Control, ably presents the main contention of the Birth Control advocates as follows:

"We believe that under any conditions, and particularly under our present economic conditions, human beings should be able to control the number of our offspring. **They should be able to decide how many children they want to have, and when they want to have them.** And to accomplish this result we demand that the knowledge of controlling the number of offspring, in other and plainer words, the knowledge of preventing undesirable conception, should not be considered criminal knowledge, that its dissemination should not be considered a criminal offense punishable by hard labor in Federal prisons, but that it should be considered knowledge useful and necessary to the welfare of the race and of the individual; and that its dissemination should be permissible and as respectable as is the dissemination of any hygienic, sanitary or eugenic knowledge.

"There is no element of force in our teachings; that is, we would not force any family to limit the number of children against their will, though we would endeavor to create a public opinion which would consider it a disgrace for any family to have more children than they can bring up and educate properly. We would consider it a disgrace, an anti-social act, for any family to bring children into the world which they must send out at an early age into the mills, shops, and streets to earn a living, or must fall back upon public charity to save them from starvation.

"Public opinion is stronger than any laws, and in time people would be as much ashamed of having children whom they could not bring up properly in every sense of the word, as they are now ashamed of having their children turn out criminals. Now, no disgrace can attach to any poor family, no matter how many children they have, because they have not got the knowledge, because society prevents them from having the knowledge of how to limit the number of children. But if that knowledge became easily accessible, and people still refused to avail themselves of it, then they would properly be considered as anti-social, as criminal members of society. As far as couples are concerned who are well-to-do, who love children, and who are well capable of taking care of a large number, we, that is, we American limitationists, would put no limit. On the contrary, we would say: 'God bless you, have as many children as you want to; there is plenty of room yet for all of you.'"

Another writer, a celebrated English thinker along these lines, has said of the general argument in favor of Birth Control:

"It used to be thought that small families were immoral. We now begin to see that it was the large families of old which were immoral. The excessive birth-rate of the early industrial period was directly stimulated by selfishness. There were no laws against child-labor; children were produced that they might be sent out, when little more than babies, to the factories and the mines to increase their parents' incomes. The diminished birth-rate has accomplished higher moral transformation. It has introduced a finer economy into life, diminished death, disease, and misery. It is indirectly, and even directly, improving the quality of the race. The very fact that children are born at longer intervals is not only beneficial to the mother's health, and therefore to the children's general welfare, but it has been proved to have a marked and prolonged influence on the physical development of children.

"Social progress, and a higher civilization, we thus see, involve **a reduced birth-rate and a reduced death-rate**. The fewer the children born, the fewer the risks of death, disease, and misery to the children that are born. The fact that civilization involves small families is clearly shown by the tendency of the educated and upper social classes to have small families. As the proletariat class becomes educated and elevated, disciplined to refinement and to foresight—as it were aristocratised—it also has small families. Civilizational progress is here on a line with biological progress. The lower organisms spawn their progeny in thousands, the higher mammals produce but one or two at a time. The higher the race, the fewer the offspring.

"Thus diminution in quantity is throughout associated with augmentation in quality. Quality rather than quantity is the racial ideal now set before us, and it is an ideal which, as we are beginning to learn, it is possible to cultivate, both individually and socially. That is why the new science of eugenics or racial hygiene is acquiring so immense an importance. In the past, racial selection has been carried out crudely by the destructive, wasteful, and expensive method of elimination, through death. In the future, it will be carried out far more effectively by conscious and deliberate selection, exercised not merely before birth, but before conception and even before mating. Galton, who recognized the futility of mere legislation to elevate the race, believed that the hope of the future lay in eugenics becoming a part of religion. The good of the race lies, not in the production of a super-man, but of a super-humanity. This can only be attained through personal individual development, the increase of knowledge, the sense of responsibility toward the race, enabling men to act in accordance with responsibility. **The leadership in civilization belongs not to the nation with the highest birth-rate, but to the nation which has thus learnt to produce the finest men and women.**"

Let us now proceed to a consideration of the special arguments in favor of rational and scientific Birth Control as advanced by its leading advocates.

The advocates of rational and scientific Birth Control have presented the strongest points of their case in their replies to those opposing the general idea, and without positively taking the stand that the burden of the proof in the argument concerning Birth Control rested upon those opposing the idea, have practically assumed that position. They claim that the right to Birth Control is so self-evident, and its application so generally recognized (though usually sought to be smothered with silence) that the case in favor of Birth Control is really quite apparent to anyone seriously considering the same without prejudice. The opposing side of the question is held by them to be represented principally by statements based on prejudice and disingenuous statements, which are capable of being turned against those advancing them.

And, the present writer, likewise is of the opinion that the strongest possible case for Birth Control is presented in the answer to the arguments advanced by the opponents thereof. But, before proceeding to the latter phase of the argument, it may be well to examine briefly the several leading points of argument advanced by the advocates of rational and scientific Birth Control, in order to clear the way for the answers to the opposite side of the question. The reader is, therefore, invited to consider the said points, briefly presented in the following paragraphs:

Birth Control Encourages Marriage. The advocates of Birth Control hold that a scientific knowledge of contraception would speedily result in a large increase of marriages, particularly among persons of limited incomes.

Persons who have not been able to accumulate the "little nest egg" which prudent persons consider a requisite on the part of those contemplating marriage and the responsibilities of rearing a family of children, are in many cases caused to hesitate about contracting marriage, and often relinquish the idea altogether. Many of these persons are well adapted for marriage, being of the domestic temperament and having the home ideal prominent in their mental makeup.

The increasing number of bachelors and unmarried women past thirty years of age, who are in evidence in all large centers of population at the present time, is undoubtedly due to a great extent to the fear on the part of these men and women regarding the proper support of a family of children. Many men and women feel that the man is able to earn enough to support himself and wife comfortably, by the exercise of economy, but that the said earnings are not sufficient to provide properly for a family of children. Some would be willing to have one or two children, born after the couple have well established themselves, but are appalled at the thought of bringing into the world a practically unlimited number of little children for whom they would not be able to provide properly.

These people shrink at the idea of abortion, and doubt the efficacy of the popular so-called contraceptive methods of which their friends tell them, and they either defer the marriage until later in life, or else give up the idea altogether as being impossible for them under the existing circumstances. A scientific knowledge of the subject would give to such persons—and there are many thousands of such—an assurance of their ability to safely and properly control and regulate the size of their families, and would lead to many a marriage which would otherwise be out of the question.

If it is agreed that the marriage state is the one normal to the average man and woman, and that marriages are in the interests of society—and few would seek to dispute this—then it would seem that anything that would tend to encourage marriage among the right kind of persons should receive the encouragement of society and be fully protected by the laws of society; and that the old prejudice against the subject, and the laws which discourage the same, and place a penalty upon the dissemination of scientific methods leading to the said result, are unworthy of civilized society and modern thought.

Earlier Marriages and Curb on Prostitution. It is generally conceded by students of sociology that earlier marriages tend to decrease the causes of the evil of prostitution, illicit sexual relations, and general sexual morality; and the consequent spread and existence of the venereal diseases which have followed in the trail of such relations. And it is likewise conceded that prostitution is an evil, and a cancer spot upon modern social life, and that venereal diseases constitute a frightful menace to the health and physical welfare of the race. Therefore, it would seem that anything which would promote early marriages among healthy, intelligent young men and women would be a blessing to the race and to society. And as these earlier marriages are unquestionably prevented in a great number of cases by reasons of the fear of inadequate financial support for large families of children, it would seem to follow that the best interests of society would be served by the encouragement by public opinion, under the protection of the law, of the teaching by competent authorities upon the subject of rational and scientific methods of Birth Control.

Health of Wives. The advocates of Birth Control lay considerable stress upon the fact that a scientific knowledge of Birth Control would practically obviate the state of broken-down health so common among married women, particularly among those who have been compelled to bear large numbers of children during the first few years of married life. Many a young married woman is in bad health—often reaching the state of chronic invalidism—as the result of having had to bear too many children, and in too close succession.

Not only is the above the case, but there is to be found on all sides many cases of invalidism and shattered health caused by the horrible practice of criminal abortion. It is doubted whether anyone outside of medical circles can even faintly begin to realize the frequency of this practice of abortion among the well-to-do, and those in "comfortable circumstances"—not to speak of the countless deaths which arise from the prevalence of this curse. Were a physician to even faintly indicate the number of cases coming under his personal professional attention, in which the patient is suffering from the effects of one or more abortions, he would be accused of gross exaggeration, and would be condemned as a sensationalist.

Without going into detail concerning these things, the writer states that it is a matter of common knowledge among physicians that in every large city there are thousands of unscrupulous (including those who call themselves physicians) who are kept busy every week in the year performing criminal operations designed to produce abortions. Some of these practitioners have many regular patients—women who visit them regularly for the purpose of having abortions produced by criminal operations. It seems almost incredible, but it is a veritable fact, that there are to be found many women in the large cities who actually boast to their friends of the number of operations of this kind they have had performed on them.

Surely, any instruction which would prevent the physical breakdown of so many women by reason of excessive child-bearing on the one hand, and abortion on the other hand, would seem to be worthy of the hearty support of society, and the encouragement of its laws, rather than the reverse. So true does this seem, that it is difficult to realize that there are any intelligent persons who would condemn such instruction as evil and harmful to society. That such persons do exist is a striking proof of the persistence of ancient superstitions and the survival and tenacity of old prejudices.

Morality of Married Men. It is a matter of common knowledge among physicians, and students of sociology, that many married men, particularly those living in the large cities, indulge in extra-marital or illicit sexual relations, with prostitutes and other women of loose morals, and this not because these men are naturally vicious, depraved or licentious, but rather because they fear causing their wives to bear them more children—the wives either being in delicate or broken-down health, or else the family already too large to be reared properly in justice to the children.

Many persons who would see only what "ought to be," and who refuse to see "things as they are" in modern society, will be disposed to pooh-pooh the above statement, and to accuse those making it to be sensational or even morbid on the subject. But those who are brought in close contact with men and women, as are family physicians and specialists, as well as honest students of sociology, know only too well that the above is not an over-statement, but is rather a very conservative recital of certain unpleasant, but true, facts of human society.

Justice to the Children. The advocates of scientific Birth Control hold that a scientific knowledge along the lines favored by them would prevent the gross injustice to children which is now only too obvious to anyone who candidly considers the matter without prejudice. The child brought into the world, unwanted, undesired, unprepared for, and unprovided for before and after birth, is handicapped from the very start of its existence upon earth. The present state of affairs works a terrible injustice upon countless children brought into the world in such conditions. Nothing that the present writer could put into words would state this fact more concisely and clearly than the following statement made by Dr. Wm. J. Robinson, a leading authority along these lines, who has said:

"The responsibility of bringing a child into the world under our present social and economic conditions is a very great one. The primitive savage or the coarse ignorant man does not care. It does not bother him what becomes of his offspring; if they get an education, if they have enough to eat, if they learn a trade or a profession, well—if they don't, also well; if they achieve a competence or a decent social position, he is satisfied—if not, he can't help it. God willed it so. But, on the other hand, the cultured, refined man and woman look at the matter differently. The thought of bringing into the world a human being which may be physically handicapped, which may be mentally inferior, which may have a hard struggle through life, which may have to go through endless misery and suffering, fills them with anguish. * * * * *

"We see about us millions of working men and women who go through life, from cradle to grave, without a ray of joy, without anything that makes life worth living. In the higher classes we see a constant, hard, infuriated struggle to make a living, to make a career, and the spectre of poverty is almost as unremittingly before the eyes of the middle and professional classes as it is before the eyes of the laborer. And all over we see ignorance, superstition, beliefs bordering on insanity, hardness, coarseness, rowdyism, brutality, crime and prostitution; prostitution of the body, and what is worse, prostitution of the mind, the hiding or selling of one's convictions for a mess of pottage. And our prisons, asylums, and hospitals are not decreasing, but increasing in number and inmates.

"It is my sincerest and deepest conviction that we could accomplish incomparably more if only a small part of the energy and money now spent on philanthropic efforts were expended in teaching the women, the married women of the poor, how to limit the number of their children; in other words, how to prevent conception. It would work a wonderful reform in the lives of the poor, and our slums would be metamorphosed in ten years. * * * It is we who are to blame now for the large families of the poor, and for this reason we are morally obligated to give them the financial and medical aid that they demand. But when effectual means are put into their hands for limiting the number of their offspring, then they, and not we, will be to blame if they do not make use of them. * * * *

"The rich and the upper-middle classes, those to whom several children would be the least burden, are quite familiar with the various means of prevention. The poorer middle classes use preventives recommended by their friends; these preventives sometimes succeed, sometimes fail, and sometimes ruin the woman's health. While the very poor, the wage-earners, those who can least afford to have unlimited progeny, knowing no means of prevention, go on breeding to their own and to the community's detriment. The result, as you can plainly see, is a general lowering of the physical and mental stamina of the race. For if the cultured and the well-to-do do not breed, or have only a few children, while the poor and the ignorant go on having a numerous progeny for which they cannot well provide, and which they cannot afford to educate properly, it stands to reason that the percentage of the uneducated, the unfit and the criminal, must go on constantly increasing. And this is something that no lover of humanity can look upon with equanimity."

Surely the above recited special points of argument in favor of Birth Control seem to be statements of self-evident facts to the unprejudiced mind, do they not? And the person of this kind who considers them carefully for the first time usually finds himself wondering what rational argument can be fairly urged on the other side of this important question. And, when he acquaints himself with the arguments of "the other side" he usually finds himself even more established in the belief that scientific Birth Control is advisable, sane, and along the lines of the mental evolution of the race. At any rate, it is difficult to escape the conviction that the burden of proof needed to controvert a proposition so nearly self-evident as intelligent and scientific Birth Control, must be placed squarely upon the shoulders of those opposing the proposition.

LESSON XIII
THE ARGUMENT AGAINST BIRTH CONTROL

The argument against Birth Control, urged by those who are opposed to the dissemination of scientific information on the subject, may be reduced to a few general points. These points of objection I shall now state, together with the rejoinder to each as given by the advocates of the proposition. I think that these points cover the main argument advanced against Birth Control, and I shall endeavor to state them as fully and as fairly as possible.

Opposed to Religious Teachings. One of the most common arguments advanced against Birth Control is the one which holds that the idea is opposed to religious teachings. The statement, however, is usually made in a vague general way, the charge of "irreligious" being hurled without explanation, and usually without any attempt to show any proof of the accusation.

As a matter of fact, as the advocates of Birth Control have pointed out, there is nothing whatsoever in the New Testament which in fairness may be construed as indicating Birth Control as sinful; in fact, it has been frequently asserted by authorities on the subject that there is nothing to be found in either the Old Testament or the New Testament which directly or indirectly prohibits the limitation of offspring, or which encourages the production of an unlimited number of children regardless of all other conditions.

Nor do the majority of the various religious denominations seem to have in their statements of doctrine and living anything in the nature of prohibition along the lines indicated above. It is true, however, that the Roman Catholic Church does quite positively, and vigorously, condemn and prohibit the use of contraceptive methods among its members; and I have been informed that its priests place such methods in the category of methods producing abortion, both being regarded as practically identical with infanticide. I have been informed, however, that in this Church the restriction of marital relations to certain periods of the month in which conception is held to be not so likely to be effected, with abstinence at other periods, is a method of limiting offspring that does not come under the ban, particularly if there be a reasonable excuse offered for the desire to limit the size of the family; though, as a rule, even such method is frowned upon unless the reasonable excuse be forthcoming.

In the case of members of the Catholic Church—and these only—there may seem to be warrant for the objection to Birth Control as "contrary to religion," it being assumed that the teachings and rules of the Church constitute the true measure of "religion." To such there is, of course, only one answer, and that is that if the teaching or practice of Birth Control methods be held by them to be "contrary to religion" (according to their definition of "religion") then they have merely to adhere to the said religious teachings, and to refuse to learn anything about Birth Control. The matter undoubtedly is one entirely for the exercise of their own judgment and conscience. There is no desire on the part of the advocates of Birth Control to insist that such people must limit the size of their families—or for that matter that there is any "must" about it for anyone whatsoever.

But we must not lose sight of the fact that the laws and customs of society in general are not based upon, or bound up with, the teachings and rules of this particular Church. On the contrary, particularly in the instance of Marriage and Divorce, many of our customs sanctioned by our laws permit and sanction things which are not countenanced or approved of by the Church in question. But just as persons outside of that Church are in no way bound by the teachings or rules thereof in the matter of Marriage and Divorce, so are they in no way bound by the teachings and rules of the said Church concerning the limitation of the size of families. The Church in question does not regard "civil marriages" as true marriages at all—yet our laws, and general public opinion, countenance such marriages; and it is extremely probable that within a comparatively short time the status of Birth Control will likewise manifest the same conflict between State and Church. But just as no Catholic is **compelled** to accept or practice civil marriage, so no Catholic will be compelled to accept or practice Birth Control.

Religion is entirely a matter of individual belief and faith, and binds no one not agreeing with its precepts. There is no union of Church and State in this country, or in most other modern civilized countries; and we are not under the jurisdiction of the Church in matters of conscience or conduct, unless we voluntarily so place ourselves under such jurisdiction and control. The argument that Birth Control which is based upon the assertion that it is opposed to the edicts or dogmas of some particular Church organization, is found to be no true argument for the reasons given above; and such argument must be dismissed as fallacious by those who base their judgments and conduct upon the dictates of science, reason, and common-sense, rather than upon the dogmas or decrees of any Church organization. The answer to those who urge that "Birth Control is contrary to the teachings of the Catholic Church" is: "Well, what of it? if you are not a Catholic!"

The force of the above objection to Birth Control becomes important when we find that those who are opposed to Birth Control merely because their Church condemns it do not content themselves with letting alone the subject, but would also endeavor to fasten the rule of their Church upon the rest of society. While such persons are undoubtedly acting in good faith, and inspired by motives which seem good to them, they should stop to remember that general society refuses to accept the rules of their Church in the matter of Marriage and Divorce, and is likely to refuse a like attempt to fasten upon it the rules of the Church in the case of Birth Control. The general public, here and in the first mentioned cases, will insist upon entering a plea of "**lack of jurisdiction**."

In the cases of persons outside of the Church in question who may consider Birth Control to be contrary to their religious convictions and teachings, there is to be made the same answer given above, namely, that the advocates of Birth Control are not trying to force anything upon those who entertain such religious or conscientious scruples—they would leave such persons free to follow the dictates of their own conscience or the religious teachings favored by them. But at the same time they would demand the legal and moral right to follow the dictates of their own conscience and reason, and would insist upon their right to receive legal protection for the dissemination of their scientific teachings. All that the advocates of Birth Control are claiming is the right of free speech and free knowledge concerning this subject which they deem concerned with the future progress and well-being of the race.

The argument against Birth Control which is based upon the claim that it is "irreligious," arises from the general tradition based upon the Hebrew conception of a Deity who bade the legendary first families of the race to "increase and multiply." According to the scriptural narrative this authoritative command was addressed to a world inhabited by eight people. From such a point of view a world's population of a few thousand persons would have seemed inconceivably great. But the old legendary command has become a tradition which has survived amid conditions totally unlike those under which it arose.

Under this old traditionary conception reproduction was regarded as a process in which men's minds and wills had no part. To those holding it, knowledge of Nature was still too imperfect for the recognition of the fact that the whole course of the world's natural history has been an erection of barrier against wholesale and indiscriminate reproduction. Thus it came about that under the old dispensation, which is now forever passing away, to have as many children as possible and to have them as often as possible —providing that certain ritual prescriptions were fulfilled—seemed to be a religious duty.

Today the conditions have altogether altered, and even our own feelings have altered. We no longer feel with the ancient Hebrew who bequeathed his ideals, though not his practices, to Christendom, that to have as many wives and concubines and as large a family as possible is both natural and virtuous and in the best interests of religion. We realize, moreover, that such claimed Divine Commands were the expression of the prophets and rulers of the people to whom they were addressed, and in accordance with the ideals concerning race-betterment which were held by these self-constituted authorities.

To the educated men and women of today, it is seen that these ideals of human-betterment (no longer imposed upon the people under the guise of Divine Commands, but rather by an appeal to their reason and judgment) are no longer based upon the sanctification of the impulse of the moment, but rather involve restraint of the impulse of the moment as taught by the lessons of foresight and regard for the future which the race has received. We no longer believe that we are divinely ordered to be reckless, or that God commands us to have children who, as we ourselves know, are fatally condemned to disease or premature death. Matters which we formerly believed to be regulated only by Providence, are now seen to be properly regulated by the providence, prudence, foresight, and self-restraint of men themselves. These characteristics are those of moral men, and those persons who lack these characteristics are condemned by our social order to be reckoned among the dregs of mankind. Our social order is one in which the sphere of procreation could not be reached or maintained by the systematic control of offspring.

More and more is Religion perceived to be more than a mere matter of the observance of certain ritual and ceremonies, or the belief in certain dogmas. More and more is true religion seen to be vitally concerned and bound up with the relations of man to man, and the welfare of society in general. More and more is it being perceived that anything which is decidedly anti-social, or opposed to the best interests of human-betterment, is not truly "religious," no matter how sanctified by tradition, or bound up with ritual and ceremonies it may be.

The spirit of modern Christianity is seen to consist of two fundamental principles, viz.: (1) the love of God; and (2) the Golden Rule. The conscientious Christian who uses head and heart in harmony and unison, cannot avoid the conclusion that the avoidance of the bringing into the world of offspring destined by social and economic conditions to misery, poverty, and sin, is more in accordance with the true spirit of Christianity than opposed to it—the ancient dogmas and traditions of the Church to the contrary notwithstanding. Modern religion is based upon Reason as well as upon Faith, and it is safe to predict the time when Birth Control will not only be sanctioned by "religion," but also encouraged by it.

Is It Immoral? Akin to the objection urged against Birth Control on the score of conflict with religious teachings, we find the one which states that "it is **immoral**." Morality means "quality of an action which renders it right or good; right conduct." Right conduct or "good" action depends upon the effect of the conduct or action upon the individual, other individuals, or society in general. The standards of morality, right conduct, and good actions have changed from time to time in the history of the race, and are not fixed. Reason teaches that that which is for the benefit of the individual and the race is and must be "moral," and that which is harmful to the individual and the race is and must be "immoral."

As to whether Birth Control is helpful or harmful to the individual and the race—moral or immoral—the individual student of the question must decide for himself after having given the subject careful and unprejudiced consideration. The advocates of Birth Control hold that every fair argument and consideration of the question must bring the unprejudiced person to the conviction that the ideals advanced by them are in the direction of the betterment of the race, and the increased happiness of the individuals composing the race. If such be the case, then Birth Control must be regarded as positively "moral" in character and principles, and its teachings directly in the interests of "morality."

So true is the above statement that every argument of the advocates of Birth Control is based upon the assumption of its "morality," in the sense of making for human betterment. If it be shown that the teachings are in anywise "immoral," in the sense indicated, then no one would be quicker to condemn them than the intelligent and conscientious advocate of Birth Control, for the reason that his whole case is based upon the inherent "morality" of his ideals.

Any one who has made a careful and unprejudiced study of the subject of Birth Control will discard the idea that a tendency so deeply rooted in Nature as is Birth Control can ever be in opposition to morality. It can only be so held as contrary to morality when men confuse the eternal principles of morality, whatever they may be, with their temporary applications, which are always becoming modified in adaptation to changing circumstances.

The old ideals of morality placed the whole question of procreation under the authority (after God) of men. Women were in subjection to men, and had no right of freedom, no right to responsibility, no right to knowledge, for, it was believed, if they were entrusted with any of these they would abuse them at once. This view prevails even today in some civilized countries, and middle-aged Italian parents, for instance, will not allow their daughters to be conducted by a man even to Mass, for they believe that as soon as they are out of their sight they will be unchaste. That is their morality.

Our morality today is different. It is inspired by different ideas, and aims at a different practice. We are by no means disposed to rate highly the morality of a girl who is only chaste so long as she is under her parents' eyes; for us, indeed, that is much more like immorality than morality. We, today, wish women to be reasonably free; we wish them to be trained in a sense of responsibility for their own actions; we wish them to possess knowledge, more especially in the sphere of sex, once theoretically opposed to them, which we now recognize as peculiarly their own domain.

Our ideal woman today is not she who is deprived of freedom and knowledge in the cloister, even though only the cloister of her own home; but rather the woman who being instructed from early life in the facts of sexual physiology and sexual hygiene, is also trained to exercise judgment, will, self-restraint, and self-responsibility, and able and worthy to be trusted to follow the path which is right according to the highest ideals of the society of which she is a part. That is the only kind of morality which now seems to us to be worth while.

And, as any unprejudiced intelligent person is forced to admit, there is nothing in the policy of scientific Birth Control to run contrary to such an ideal of moral womanhood.

But the relation of Birth Control to morality is, however, by no means a question which concerns women alone. It equally concerns men. Here we have to recognize, not only that the exercise of control over procreation enables a man to form a marriage of faithful devotion with the woman of his choice at an earlier age than would otherwise be possible, but it further enables him, throughout the whole of his married life, to continue such relationship under circumstances which might otherwise render them injurious or else undesirable to his wife.

That the influence exerted by a general knowledge of scientific methods of Birth Control would suffice to entirely abolish prostitution it is foolish to maintain, although it would undoubtedly tend to decrease the social evil. And even the partial elimination of prostitution would be in the interests of general morality, not only in the direction of lessening the brutal demand of women to serve in the ranks of prostitution, but also in many other ways of importance to society as a whole. The decrease of venereal disease would follow a decrease in prostitution caused by a general knowledge and practice of scientific methods of Birth Control on the part of married people; and it must be remembered that venereal disease spreads far beyond the patrons of prostitution and is a perpetual menace to others who may become innocent victims. And any influence that serves to decrease prostitution and the spread of venereal disease, must be placed in the category of "moral," and certainly not in the opposite one.

The objection is frequently heard that the general knowledge of scientific methods of contraception would lead to increased illicit relations among unmarried persons, particularly among the young people. This argument is apparently based upon the belief, or fear, that the fear of conception is the only thing which prevents many persons from indulging in illicit relations. It assumes that a large portion of our womankind are chaste simply because of fear of pregnancy; and that this fear once removed these women would at once plunge into such relations. In other words, it assumes that mentally and in spirit these women are already unchaste, but are restrained from physical unchastity by reason of the fear of conception.

The answer of the advocates of Birth Control takes direct issue with the above contention. On the contrary, it asserts that the chastity of our women is the result of their general training, education, heredity, observance of the accepted customs and standards of their community, religious and moral training, etc. The woman who is chaste simply through fear, usually manages to allay that fear in one way or another, often by mistaken methods which work great harm to the woman and the community in general. The general knowledge of scientific contraceptive methods might result in such women manifesting their inclinations and desires in a "safer" manner, but this "safety" would not consist of protection against conception (for that they already think they have) but rather of a protection against the dangers of abortion and similar evil practices.

Some of the writers go further in this matter, as for instance Dr. Robinson, who says: "If some women are bound to have illicit relations, is it not better that they should know the use of scientific preventives than that they should become pregnant, disgracing and ostracising themselves, and their families;

or that they should subject themselves to the degradation and risks of an abortion; or failing this, take carbolic acid or bichloride, jump into the river, or throw themselves under the wheels of a running train?"

The objection to Birth Control on the ground that it would increase illicit relations among men and women by means of removing the fear of physical consequences, seems to many careful thinkers to be akin to the old objection (now happily passing away) to the dissemination of the knowledge of the treatment of venereal diseases, and to the public cure of such diseases, on the ground that by so doing a part of the fear concerning illicit relations was removed, and thereby illicit relations actually encouraged. The result of this fallacious argument was the enormous spread of venereal diseases, to the great hurt of the race; and the encouragement of quacks and charlatans who fattened on the gains received from the sufferers from this class of complaints. The argument against Birth Control on similar grounds will be seen to be equally fallacious, and capable of equally evil consequences, if the matter be fairly and carefully considered.

Illicit relations, if prevented or regulated at all by society, must be so regulated or prevented by other means than fear of conception. Such fear, though it may deter for a short time, will usually be overcome in time if the desire and temptation remain sufficiently strong. It is doubtful whether any considerable number of women remain chaste for any length of time simply by reason of fear of conception. If such fear be the only remaining deterring factor, it will usually be swept away in time under continued temptation, opportunity, and desire. Chastity and virtue must have a far more solid foundation than such fear; and experience repeatedly shows that such fear is but as shifting sand sought to be employed as a foundation for the structure of chastity.

There is no reason whatsoever for believing that the scientific knowledge of contraceptive methods, if generally possessed by married people under the sanction of the law and society, would result in any more cases of illicit relations than exist at the present time. It might, it is true, result in less evil consequences of such relations in some cases, as Dr. Robinson has so clearly pointed out in the above quotation; but the relations in such cases would exist in either event. Fear of conception, like fear of infection, has never, and will never entirely prevent illicit relations between men and women; and to oppose scientific information in the one case on these grounds, is as futile as to oppose scientific treatment in the other case on the same grounds. And when it is considered how society in general is injured by the withholding of such information or treatment, respectively, the argument in favor of such suppression of scientific truth and method is seen to be actually dangerous to society and sub-service of the public good.

I would like to add a few words concerning the question of morality in the matter of practicing scientific Birth Control. To me what I shall say in the succeeding paragraphs of this chapter have a vital bearing on the whole subject, and should be taken into serious consideration by the fair-minded and conscientious student of the subject. Here follows my thought in the matter:

In my consideration of the arguments against scientific Birth Control I am impressed with one particular thought which refuses to be silenced, but which insists upon persistently presenting itself to my consciousness. This particular thought may be expressed as follows: It is admitted by unprejudiced students of the subject that the educated and cultured portions of the civilized countries of modern times do actually practice, to some extent, in some form, manner, or degree, the limitation of offspring—no honest observer will dispute this statement. This being so, does it not seem that the race should fairly and squarely, honestly and frankly, face this question and decide whether or not such rules of conduct are "right" or "wrong"—"moral" or "immoral"—and to what extent, if any, they should be permitted or encouraged to be practiced toward the ends of individual and race happiness and betterment.

If the decision is totally against this rule of conduct, then it should be vigorously denounced, and all honest people should refrain from it. If, on the contrary, the decision should be that this mode of conduct, or some phases of it, are justified, then, in the name of Honesty and Truth, let us turn on the full light of general information, knowledge, and instruction on the subject, under the full protection of the laws and public opinion. Why should we not throw aside the mask of cowardly hypocrisy, and stand before the world showing ourselves as just what we really are?

My thought, in essence, is that the chief "wrong," and "immorality" about the whole matter consists in our present practice of doing one thing in private, and condemning the same thing in public. There can be no excuse, to the intellectually honest person at least, for the course of tacitly holding that a certain thing is "all right for us," while "all wrong for the other folks."

Is It Injurious to Health? It is sometimes urged against Birth Control that the use of contraceptive methods is injurious to the health of women, in some cases a long list of physical and mental ills being given as possible of being caused by such methods. Opposed to this is the contention of the members of the medical profession who have arrayed themselves on the side of scientific Birth Control. The latter authorities positively contradict the assertion that women's health is injured by the practice of rational and scientific methods of Birth Control; although these authorities freely admit, in fact they **claim**, that certain unscientific methods and practices popular among certain persons—such as the use of certain chemicals and mechanical appliances—undoubtedly have resulted in physical harm, and they strongly advise against the use of such bunglesome methods.

One of the leading medical advocates of scientific Birth Control in the United States throws down the gauntlet squarely before those of his profession, and others, who urge this objection to scientific Birth Control, in the following challenging words: "I challenge any physician, any gynecologist, to bring forth **a single authenticated case** in which disease or injury resulted from the use of modern methods of prevention. I know they cannot do it." And others in the ranks of the medical profession have made similar assertions and claims. The unprejudiced person who will consult the best medical authorities on the subject will unquestionably agree that the best medical opinion of the day holds that scientific Birth Control is not in fairness to be open to this objection.

Is Birth Control Unnatural? Another favorite argument of the opponents of scientific Birth Control is the broad statement and claim that "all voluntary attempts to limit procreation are unnatural," and therefore wrong. This objection, while usually offered without any particular argument, explanation, or proof, must be carefully and honestly met and answered by the fair-minded advocate of Birth Control.

In the first place, it may as well be admitted that regulation, restriction, or control of the procreative functions by application of the intellect or reasoning processes **is** unnatural, in the sense of not being indicated by Nature and enforced through the instinctive actions of the race. The only instinct which primitive man seems to have had in this case (and these he held in common with the lower animals) was that of free and unlimited sexual intercourse, in response to his instinctive desires, with this exception (and this exception should be carefully noted), i. e.: that the male respected the instinctive disinclination to cohabit during the period in which the woman was pregnant, and often also during the period in which she nursed her infant. This instinct, unhappily for the race, the "civilized" man has overridden until it has practically ceased to manifest its voice.

The lower animals, obeying this primitive instinct, do not manifest violation of this law of Nature. On the contrary, the female will not allow the male to approach her at such times, and will fight savagely at any attempt to violate this instinctive law of her nature. The male usually recognizes the existence of this law, and makes no attempt to violate it, but should he attempt the same he is defeated by the female as above stated. It has remained for Man alone to override and violate, and to eventually render nul and void this wise instinctive provision of Nature.

But beyond this there is no "natural," instinctive regulation of the sexual activities of animal or man, other than the desires of the male and female. If civilized man adhered wholly to the "natural" in this respect, he would obey the voice of instinct alone, and would show reason and intellect the door in such matters, and would also bid defiance to all legal or ecclesiastical authority when it sought to "control" his activities along these lines. But, it is needless to say, such is not the case. Not only has the Law of the Church insisted upon certain "control" of these matters—as witness the laws against adultery, illicit relations, incest, bastardy, etc.—but man, himself, has asserted a greater and still greater voluntary control over the reproductive functions as he has risen in the scale of civilization and culture.

Today it is only the lowest and least cultured classes of society who (to use the expressive but somewhat inelegant term) persist in "breeding like pigs." All other classes exercise a greater or less degree of "control" of some kind in the matter of limitation of offspring. In making this broad assertion I, of course, have in mind not only the modern methods urged by the advocates of scientific contraception, but also the "control" and regulation observed by married persons in either total abstinence from the marital relations for a stated time, or else the abstinence from such relations during certain portions of the lunar month, the latter method (somewhat uncertain, however, in its efficacy in some cases) being apparently favored by certain ecclesiastical authorities as the "only moral" method.

In view of the above facts, which might be enlarged and extended if necessary, it is seen that as soon as man rises above the level of the beast or savage—as soon as he begins to manifest culture and civilization—he begins to exercise a certain "control" over the procreative **function**, and in the direction of the limitation of the size of his family of offspring. The contention of the modern advocates of scientific Birth Control is that the "new ideas" on the subject are simply a natural and inevitable evolution from the degrees of "control" which man has exercised since the time he emerged from savagery. The later developments are no more "unnatural" than the earlier—nor the accepted methods and forms any more "natural" than those which are now opposed by the more conservative elements of society.

When anyone begins to talk about things being "natural" or "unnatural," respectively, he should tread softly and watch his steps carefully. For at every step he treads upon instances of "unnatural" modes and methods of living. Strictly speaking, it is "unnatural" to wear clothes, or to cook food, or to live in houses, or to ride in conveyances or on horseback. All of these things have been evolved by the use of intellect and reason, and are not instinctive or "natural" to man. Birds build nests, wasps build shelter, hornets build homes, bees build honey-combs, worms build cocoons, snails build shells—all by instinct and "naturally"—and the young of such species do not have to be **taught** how to do these things. But the young of the human race requires to be taught such things as above mentioned as having been evolved by man in the course of his rise from savagery—instinct will not do it for them. And all of these things outside the plane of instinct, and within the plane of intellect, cannot be called "natural" in the strict sense of the term.

You think that I am exaggerating the matter, perhaps. Well, then, I ask you to consider the meaning of the two terms which I have employed so freely in the foregoing paragraphs: First, let us consider the term, "**Natural**"; we find it defined as "**fixed or determined by nature, and, therefore, according to nature, and not artificial, assumed, or acquired**." Next, let us consider the term, "**Instinct**"; we find it defined as "**natural impulse, or unconscious, involuntary, or unreasoning prompting to any action**." It will be seen, accordingly, that merely the most elemental and primitive activities of man are "natural" in this sense; and that all his acquired activities and methods are "not natural."

The activities of man which are in the "not natural" class may be either desirable for the individual and the race, or else undesirable for both. Therefore, it will be seen, all such activities must be subjected to the test of reason and experience in order to determine whether they are in the best interests of the individual and the race, or else opposed to these. This is the only sane method of testing the validity and desirability of such things— Birth Control among the others. The claim of "not natural," if applied at all, must be extended to **all** things which are not strictly "natural" or instinctive —it is casuistical to apply the term in reproach to certain things and to withhold it from others in the same general class.

LESSON XIV
RACE SUICIDE

A favorite argument of certain opponents of scientific Birth Control is that such teachings and modes of conduct tend toward Race Suicide, and the consequent weakening and final destruction of the human race by means of "bleeding it white" by draining from it its normal supply of children. Those who hold this view argue that if Birth Control methods become popular, and sanctioned by the law and public opinion, then the race will eventually die out and disappear from the face of the earth. Some vary the argument by insisting that those nations favoring Birth Control would suffer decline and gradual extinction at the hands of other nations opposed to scientific methods of regulating the number and frequency of offspring. This is a serious charge against Birth Control, which if proved would probably serve to array all right-thinking persons against it.

But the advocates of Birth Control seriously and positively controvert and deny the validity and truth of this argument. On the contrary they claim that scientific Birth Control would not only keep up the population of all countries, or any country, to a normal standard proportionate to its ability to sustain properly such population, but will also act to render that population stronger and better, physically, mentally and morally, and far more efficient in every way owing to improved quality of the stock. The first requisite is met by **the reduction of the death rate** to meet the decreasing birth-rate; and the second requisite is met by the improvement of the stock by proper rearing and training made possible by the decreased size of the average family. **Birth control serves to eliminate the waste caused by excessive infant mortality**, and to thus fully counterbalance the decreased birth rate.

The advocates of Birth Control assert that the natural instinct of parenthood, the love of children, and the desire for offspring and the perpetuation of the family name and stock, are too firmly rooted and grounded in human nature to be seriously affected by such knowledge and practice on the part of the race. They point to the fact that in many families in which intelligent modes of Birth Control are favored, and in which the size of the family has been limited to a few children, the children are, as a rule, better cared for and provided for, better reared and better educated, than in the case of families in which children are brought into the world without thought or reason, and without the possibility of proper care and rearing. Birth Control, say its advocates, will not do away with children, but will merely regulate their number to rational limits, and at appropriate intervals between births. Moreover, it is claimed, that while the birth-rate in such families may be smaller, **the death-rate is also smaller**. And, at the last, it is the number of children that **survive** that counts with the race, not those who merely are **born**.

The fact that many persons consult physicians for a cure for sterility, and go to great trouble and expense to further the bearing of children, and the fact many childless couples adopt children rather than to have a childless home, are evidence of the fact that there is no danger of the parental instinct dying out. It is the experience of physicians generally that the patients who desire information regarding scientific contraceptive methods are usually those who already have as many children as they can well take care of, and not those who wish to escape parenthood in toto.

We are constantly reminded that the size of the average family is much smaller than it was a hundred years ago—but still the race is rapidly increasing, owing to the decreased death-rate resulting from a better knowledge of hygiene and medicine. Moreover, it is positively asserted that the "old time large family" frequently had one father but several mothers— the husband marrying several times in order to replace with a new life the old wife who had broken down and died from overwork and excessive childbearing.

It is claimed that in Holland, in which Birth Control is recognized by law, and where it is legally sanctioned and even encouraged among those who are not able to support large families, statistics show that the population is increasing more rapidly than before, owing to the decreased mortality of infants and young children arising from the better care of those who are born.

Dr. Robinson says on this point: "Here we have a whole country, Holland, in which the prevention of conception is legally sanctioned, in which the use of preventives is practically universal—and is this country dying out? On the contrary, it is increasing more rapidly than before, because we have this remarkable and gratifying phenomenon to bear in mind, that **wherever the birth-rate goes down, the death rate goes down pari passu, or even to a still greater degree**. This can be proven by statistics from almost every country in the world. For instance, in 1910 the birth-rate in Holland was 32, and the mortality 18; in 1912 the birth-rate fell to 28, but then the mortality rate fell still lower, namely to 12, so we see an actual gain in population, instead of a loss. And the physical constitution of the people has been improving * * *. And in New Zealand, where the sale of contraceptives is practically free, the birth rate is now 20, and the mortality rate is 10. Does that look like race suicide? On the contrary, there is a steady increase at the rate of ten per cent, while sickness and death of children, with their attendant economic and emotional waste, are reduced to a minimum."

Not only are the children of small families as a rule better cared for, from economic reasons easy to discern, but it is also a fact that the health of the mothers is far better, and consequently the health of the children when born is better than the average. One has but to look around him upon the families who boast of having had eight, ten, and twelve children born to them, to see what a frightful average percentage of deaths of infants and young children is present, and which brings down the number of the survivors.

Dr. Alice Hamilton, in "The Bulletin of the American Academy of Medicine," for May, 1910, reports that she has investigated the families of 1,600 wage workers, and found the following death rate per 1,000 birth among them, viz.:

Families of 4 children and less	118 deaths per 1,000 births
Families of 6 children	267 deaths per 1,000 births
Families of 7 children	280 deaths per 1,000 births
Families of 8 children	291 deaths per 1,000 births
Families of 9 children or more	303 deaths per 1,000 births

Dr. Hamilton sums up her investigation as follows:

"Our study of the poorer working class shows that child mortality increases proportionately as the number of children increase, until we

have a death rate in families of 8 children and over which is two and a half times as great as that in families of 4 children and over."

The facts above mentioned, and other facts of the same nature which will be disclosed in the progress of our consideration of the matter in the present book, have evidently been overlooked, deliberately or otherwise, by the fanatics in this country and in Europe who have been preaching to the people that a falling birth-rate means a decaying nation. Careful students of sociology now dismiss altogether the statement so often made that a falling birth-rate means "an old and decaying community." The Germans for years have contemptuously been making this remark about France, but today they have been forced to recognize an unexpected vitality in the French, while, in fact, their own birth-rate has been falling more rapidly than that of France.

Nor is it true that a falling birth-rate means a falling population. The French birth-rate has been steadily falling for a number of years, yet the French population has been steadily increasing all the time, though less rapidly than it would had not the death-rate been abnormally high. It is not the number of babies born that counts, but the net result in surviving children. An enormous number of babies are born in China; but an enormous number die while still babies. So that it is better to have a few babies of good quality than a large number of indifferent quality, for the falling birth-rate is more than compensated by the falling death-rate. In England, as the statistics show, while the birth-rate is steadily falling, the population has been steadily growing.

Small families and a falling death-rate are not merely no evil—they are a positive good. They are a gain for humanity. They represent an evolutionary rise in Nature and a higher stage in civilization. We are here in the presence of a great fundamental principle of progress which has been working through life from the beginning.

At the beginning of life on the earth, reproduction ran riot. Of one minute organism it is estimated that, if its reproduction were not checked by death or destruction, in thirty days it would form a mass a million times larger than the sun. The conger-eel lays fifteen million eggs, and if they all grew up, and reproduced themselves on the same scale, in two years the whole sea would become a wriggling mass of eels. As we approach the higher forms of life, reproduction gradually dies down. The animals nearest to man produce few offspring, but they surround them with parental care, until they are able to lead independent lives with a fair chance of surviving. The whole process may be regarded as a mechanism for slowly subordinating quantity to quality, and to promoting the evolution of life to even higher stages.

This process, which is plain to see on the largest scale throughout living nature, may be more minutely studied, as it acts within a narrower range, in the human species. Here we statistically formulate it in the terms of birth-rate and death-rate; by the mutual relationship of the two courses of the birth-rate and death-rate we are able to estimate the evolutionary rank of a nation, and the degree in which it has succeeded in subordinating the primitive standard of quantity to the higher and later standard of quality.

Especially in Europe we can investigate this relationship by the help of statistics which in some cases extend back for nearly a century. We can trace the various phases through which each nation passes, the effects of prosperity, the influence of education and sanitary improvement, the general complex development of civilization, in each case moving forward, though not regularly and steadily, to higher stages by means of a falling birth-rate, which is to some extent compensated by a falling death-rate, the two rates nearly always running parallel, so that a temporary rise in the birth-rate is usually accompanied by a rise in the death-rate, by a return, that is to say, towards the conditions which we find at the beginning of animal life, and a steady fall in the birth-rate is always accompanied by a fall in the death-rate.

It is thus clear that the birth-rate combined with the death-rate constitutes a delicate instrument for the measurement of civilization, and that the record of their combined curves registers the upward or downward course of every nation. The curves, as we know, tend to be parallel, and when they are not parallel we are in the presence of a rare and abnormal state of things which is usually temporary or transitional.

A study of the statistics of European countries furnishes us with evidence of the facts above stated. It is instructive to perceive how closely the birth-rate and the death-rate of the several European countries agree. It is perceived that **the eight countries of Europe which register the highest birth-rate are the identical countries registering the highest death-rate**. This is as might be expected, for a very high birth-rate seems fatally to involve a very high death-rate. The study of the following table may prove interesting—it certainly is instructive. In the following table the European countries having the highest birth-rate are stated in the order of rank according to size of such rate; and the countries having the heaviest death-rate are stated in the order of their rank in size of such rate:

Highest European Birth-Rate.	*Highest European Death-Rate.*
Russia.	Russia.
Roumania.	Roumania.
Bulgaria.	Hungary.
Serbia.	Bulgaria.
Hungary.	Spain.
Italy.	Serbia.
Austria.	Austria.
Spain.	Italy.

Moreover, Japan, with a rather high birth-rate, has the same death-rate as Spain; and Chile, with a still higher birth-rate, has a higher death rate than Russia. So, we see, that among human peoples we find the same laws prevailing as among animals, and the higher nations of the world differ from those which are less highly evolved precisely as the elephant differs from the herring, though within a narrower range, that is to say, **by producing fewer offspring and taking better care of them.**

So, when we get to the root of the matter, the whole question of "Does Birth Control tend toward Race Suicide?" becomes clear, and we are able to answer, positively, "It certainly does not; on the contrary it tends toward Race Progress and Race Betterment." We see that there is really no standing ground in any country for the panic-monger who bemoans the fall of the birth-rate, and storms against small families. The falling birth-rate is a world-wide phenomenon in all countries that are striving toward a higher civilization along lines which Nature laid down from the beginning. We cannot stop it if we would, and if we could we should be merely impeding civilization. It is a movement which rights itself and tends to reach a just balance.

Instead of trying to raise the birth-rate by offering a bonus on babies as has been proposed in some quarters, it would be saner and better calculated for the betterment of the race to offer a bonus upon young men and women who attained maturity with a definite high standard of physical and mental development. As a writer on the subject has well said: "But we need not therefore fold our hands and do nothing. There is much still to be effected for the protection of motherhood and the better care of children. We cannot, and should not, attempt to increase the number of children born; there is still far more misery in having too many babies than in having too few; a bonus on babies would be a misfortune, alike for the parents and the State. **But we may well work for the better quality of babies.** There we should be on very safe ground. More knowledge is necessary so that all would-be parents may know how they may best become parents, and how they may, if necessary, best avoid it. Procreation by the unfit should be, if not prohibited by law, at all events so discouraged by public opinion that to attempt it would be considered disgraceful. Much greater public provision is necessary for the care of mothers during the months before, as well as in the period after, the child's birth. Along such lines as these we may hope to increase the happiness of the people and the strength of the State. We need not worry about the falling birth-rate."

The more that one intelligently examines the argument against Birth Control based upon fear of Race Suicide, the more one becomes convinced that not only is there "nothing to it," but that every fact brought to light in the inquiry reveals itself in the nature of proof of the desirability of Birth Control as a factor of Race Evolution, rather than evidence to the contrary.

Therefore, the more inquiry and investigation that such argument brings forth, the stronger is the case disclosed for Birth Control, and the greater the amount of public opinion created in its favor.

In all considerations of the general question of Race Suicide, one must take note of the general question of Eugenics or Human Breeding. This because the sound breeding of the race operates in a direction diametrically opposed to Race Suicide, while unsound breeding operates directly in favor thereof.

When we consider the general subject of Eugenics we touch upon the highest ground, and are concerned with our best hopes for the future of the world. There can be no doubt that Birth Control, considered as a phase of Eugenics, is not only a precious but also an indispensable instrument in moulding the coming man to the measure of our developing ideals. Without Birth Control we are powerless in the face of the awful evils which flow from random and reckless reproduction. With it we possess a power so great that some persons have professed to see in it a menace to the propagation of the race, amusing themselves with the idea that if people possess the means to prevent the conception of children they will never have children at all. It is not necessary to discuss such a grotesque notion seriously.

The desire for children is far too deeply implanted in mankind and womankind alike ever to be rooted out. If there are today many parents whose lives are rendered wretched by large families and the miseries of excessive child-bearing, there are an equal number whose lives are wretched because they have no children at all, and who snatch eagerly at any straw which offers the smallest promise of relief to the craving. Certainly there are people who desire marriage, but—some for very sound and estimable reasons and other for reasons which may less well bear examination—do not desire children at all.

For the class of married people who do not desire children at all, contraceptive methods, far from being a social evil, are a social blessing. For nothing is as certain as that it is an unmixed evil for a community to possess unwilling, undesirable parents. Birth Control would be an unmixed blessing if it merely enabled us to exclude such persons from the ranks of parenthood. We desire no parents who are not competent and willing parents. Only such parents are fit to father and to mother a future race worthy to rule the world.

It is sometimes said that the control of conception, since it is frequently carried out immediately upon marriage, will tend to delay parenthood until an unduly late age. Birth Control has, however, no necessary result of this kind, and might even act in the reverse direction. A chief cause of delay in marriage is the prospect of the burden and expense of an unrestricted flow of children into the family; and it is said that in Great Britain, since 1911, with the extension of the use of contraceptives, there has been a slight but regular increase not only in the general marriage rate but also in the proposition of early marriage. The ability to control the number of children not only enables marriage to take place at an early age, but also makes it possible for the couple to have at least one child soon after marriage. The total number of children are thus spaced out, instead of following in rapid succession.

It is only of late years that the eugenic importance of a considerable interval between births has been fully recognized, as regards not only the mother—this has long been recognized—but also the children. The very high mortality of large families has long been known, and their association with degenerate conditions and with criminality. However, of recent years, evidence has been obtained that families in which the children are separated from each other by intervals of more than two years are both mentally and physically superior to those in which the interval is shorter. Investigators have found that children born at only a short interval after the birth of a previous child are notably defective, even at the age of six, in a large percentage of cases; and when compared with children born at a longer interval, or with first children, they are, on the average, three inches shorter and three pounds lighter. These are facts of the most vital significance.

Thus when we calmly survey, in however summary a manner, the great field of life affected by the establishment of voluntary human control over the production of the race, we can not see a cause for anything but hope. It is satisfactory that it should be so, for there can be no doubt that we are here facing a great and permanent fact in civilized life. With every rise in civilization, indeed with all evolutionary progress whatever, there is what seems to be an automatic fall in the birth-rate. That fall is always normally accompanied by a fall in the death-rate, so that a low birth-rate frequently means a high rate of natural increase, since most of the children born survive.

Thus in the civilized world of today, notwithstanding the low birth-rate which prevails as compared with earlier times, the rate of increase in the population is still appalling—nearly half a million a year in Great Britain, over a million in Austro-Hungary, and three-quarters of a million in Germany. When we examine this excess of births in detail we find among them a large proportion of undesired and undesirable children. There are two alternative methods working to diminish this proportion: the method of regulating conception under the methods of scientific Birth Control, or the bungling substitutes for the same, on the one hand, and the method of preventing live births after conception by means of the abominable practice of abortion.

There can be no doubt about the enormous extension of the practice of abortion in all civilized countries, even although some of the extravagant estimates of its frequency in countries, the United States for example, be discarded as unwarranted. The burden of bearing excessive children on the overworked and underfed mothers of the working classes becomes at last so intolerable that almost anything seems better than another child. As a woman in Yorkshire once said to an English investigator of this evil: "I'd rather swallow the druggist's shop and the man in it, than have another kid."

A community which takes upon itself the responsibility of encouraging abortion lays itself open to severe criticism. And it must be admitted that just as all those who work for Birth Control are really diminishing the frequency of abortion, so every attempt to discourage Birth Control promotes abortion. We have to approach this problem calmly, in the light of Nature and reason. We have each of us to decide on which side to range ourselves. For it is a vital problem concerning which we cannot afford to be indifferent.

There is no desire here to exaggerate the importance of Birth Control. It is not a royal road to the millennium of the race; and like all other measures which the course of progress forces us to adopt, it has its disadvantages. But fairness and honest thought should admit freely that so far as is concerned the question of its being a factor toward Race Suicide, we must pronounce a verdict of "Not Guilty" upon Birth Control. On the contrary, the contrary course of teaching and practice, if carried to their full logical conclusion, would inevitably bring the race to such a stage of degeneracy, and retrogression to primitive type, that a fate far worse than suicide would befall the human race. For the race, as well as the individual, may commit "suicide" and an end to its career, not only by a will-not-to-live but also by a will-to-degenerate.

The face of Birth Control is set toward the rising sun of Race Betterment, not toward the setting sun of Racial Decline. Its ideas are those of Race Life, not of Race Death. It bids the race not to perish, but rather to live on in greater strength, happiness, and efficiency. Birth Control is in full accord with the Racial Will-to-Live, and not opposed to it. All humanity, all civilization, all human progress, call upon us to take our stand upon this vital question of Birth Control. And, as a writer has well said, in doing so we shall each of us be contributing, however humbly, to that "one far-off event, to which the whole creation moves."

LESSON XV
BIRTH CONTROL METHODS

The general subject of Birth Control necessarily includes the special subject of Birth Control Methods, viz., of the methods of association between husband and wife under which offspring is conceived only at such times as desired, and consequently only in the number desired.

These methods may be grouped into three general classes, as follows:

I. Methods of Continence (total or temporary). In the practice of the methods under this class, there is an avoidance of sexual relations between husband and wife, either continuously or for certain periods during which the liability to conception is great.

II. Methods of Semi-Continence. In the practice of the methods under this class, there is a partial manifestation of the sexual relation accompanied by an absence of the manifestation of the procreative functions.

III. Methods of Contraception. In the practice of the methods under this class, the usual manifestations of the sexual relation are observed, accompanied by an avoidance of the union of the male and female elements of reproduction which result in conception.

The student of the subject of Birth Control, of course, familiarizes himself or herself with each of the several classes of methods above noted, for the purpose of understanding the characteristic distinctions between them, and the respective advantages and disadvantages of each class. In the following pages each class will be briefly considered, that the student may acquire a general understanding thereof, and may be enabled to reason intelligently concerning them. In this presentation there will be sought a fair statement of each class, without any desire to influence the student for or against either of them.

Continence.

Continence (which in this special sense means the avoidance of sexual relations between husband and wife), in the strict sense, is based upon the idea that the sexual relation should not be exercised except for the purpose and intent of procreation. In the restricted usage of the term, it refers to the abstinence from sexual intercourse during stated periods in which the liability to conception is greatest.

Rev. Sylvanus Stall, the author of several widely-read works on the subject of Sex, says of strict continence: "One theory is that the reproductive function is not to be exercised except for the purpose of procreation. * * * There are some married people, more numerous than some suppose, who have adopted the idea of uniform continence, and who call the reproductive nature into exercise for the purpose of procreation only, and who assert that the maintenance of continence secures not only the greater strength and better health, but greater happiness also. * * * While the results of our investigations do not enable us to assert that it is the true theory, we are yet prepared to say that it is worthy of thoughtful consideration. If it is possible for married people to maintain absolute continence for a period of six months or a year, it must be conceded that it would be possible to extend that time to a longer period. The maintenance of this theory would require such a degree of self-control as is far beyond the possession of the great mass of humanity. We fear, also, that there are but few, even if they entered upon a life union with such thought and intention, who would be willing to maintain their principles for any considerable period. * * * The other theory, and that which many men and women who are eminent for their learning and religious life hold to be the correct theory, is that while no one has a right to enter upon the marriage relation with the fixed purpose of evading the duty of parenthood, yet that procreation is not the only high and holy purpose which God has had in view in establishing the marriage relation, but that the act of sexual congress may be indulged in between husband and wife for the purpose of expressing their personal endearments, and for quickening those affections and tender feelings which are calculated to render home the place of blessing and good which God intended. * * * It is held by those who advocate this theory, that while it would be possible to restrict the exercise of the reproductive functions to the single purpose of procreation, yet in the great majority of instances the effort to live by that theory would generally result in marital unhappiness. * * * Due regard is not only to be paid to the perpetuity of the race, but to the well-being and perpetuity of the individual."

The advocates of continence, except for the purpose of procreation, advance many arguments and evidence to justify their contention that this is the only course justified by Nature and Morality. We need not present this argument here, for it is outside the particular question now under consideration. However, in all fairness and justice, there should be presented here the general outline of their argument that there is no rational basis for the widely accepted idea that abstinence from sexual relations is in any way harmful or detrimental to the health and physical well-being of the human race.

The advocates of continence cite the cases of many continent men who have been noted for their vigor and activity; and claim that such cases also justify their claim that continence makes for the sound mind in the sound body of mankind. The following quotations from authorities will give the general spirit of this contention.

Dr. Kellogg says: "It has been claimed by many, even physicians, and though with but a slight show of reason, that absolute continence, after a full development of the organs of reproduction, could not be maintained without a great detriment to health. It is needless to enumerate all the different arguments employed to support this position, since they are, with a few exceptions, too frivolous to mention." Dr. Mayer says: "This position is held by men of the world, and many physicians share it. This belief appears to us erroneous, without foundation, and easily refuted. No peculiar disease nor any abridgement of the duration of life can be ascribed to such continence. * * * Health does not absolutely require that there should ever be an emission of semen, from puberty to death, though the individual live a hundred years." Dr. Kellogg also says: "This has been amply confirmed by experiments upon animals, as well as by the experience of some of the most distinguished men who have ever lived, among whom may be mentioned Sir Isaac Newton, Kant, Paschal, Fontenaille, and Michael Angelo. These men never married, and lived continent lives. Some of them lived to be a very great age, retaining to the last their wonderful abilities. In view of this fact, there is certainly no danger."

Another writer has said: "The Greek athletes training for the great Olympic Games were compelled to observe strict continence, the experience being that by this course they were able to conserve their vigor and strength much better. The prize-fighters of today are compelled by their trainers to observe strict continence during the period of training. Many of the former champions who went to pieces suddenly, owe their downfall to a violation of this rule." Another has said: "Chastity, even continence, is the prime necessity of the successful athlete." Dr. Kellogg forcefully says: "Breeders of stock who wish to secure sound progeny will not allow the most robust stallion to associate with mares as many times during the whole season as some of these salacious human males perform a similar act within a month."

Dr. Warbasse has said: "Testicular fluid in the seminal vesicles, under unexciting conditions, does not require to be discharged at intervals. I have not been able to find in the studies of the physiologists that its retention is abnormal or unhygienic. * * * I do not conceive of a man suffering from the ills of continence who has been cast away on a desert island, with no immediate prospect of relief, and whose mind and hands are occupied with raising grain, catching fish for subsistence, and constructing a boat for escape. All that has been said of men may be said of women."

Dr. Talmey has said: "Continence, if long continued, has been claimed to be the cause of impotence. But there is no valid reason for this belief. To prove the harmfulness of continence an analogue is brought forward between the atrophy of a muscle in enforced idleness and the injury to the sex organs in enforced abstinence. But the proof is somewhat feeble. The essential organs of generation are not muscles, but glands, and who has ever heard of a tear gland atrophying for lack of crying. * * * There is no valid proof of the harmfulness of total abstinence in a healthy individual. A perfectly healthy man is never injured by abstinence. At least there is no sufficient proof that he ever was; but there are unmistakable proofs that total abstinence does not harm the individual."

Dr. Stockham has said: "The testes may be considered analogous to the salivary and lachrymal glands, in which there is no fluid secreted except at the demand of their respective functions. The thought of food makes the mouth water for a short time only, while the presence of food causes abundant yield of saliva. It is customary for physicians to assume that the spermatic secretion is analogous to bile, which, when once formed, must be expelled. But substitute the word 'tears' for bile, and you put before the mind an idea entirely different. Tears, as falling drops, are not essential to life and health. A man may be in perfect health and yet not cry once in five or even fifty years. The lachrymal fluid is ever present, but in such small quantities that it is unnoticed. Where are tears while they remain unshed? They are ever ready, waiting to spring forth when there is an adequate cause, but they do not accumulate and distress the man because they are not shed daily, weekly, or monthly. The component elements of the tears are prepared in the system, they are on hand, passing through the circulation, ready to mix and flow whenever they are needed; but if they mix, accumulate and flow without adequate cause, there is a disease of the lachrymal glands. While there are no exact analogies in the body, yet the tears and the spermatic fluids are much more closely analogous in their normal manner of secretion and use than are the bile and the semen. Neither flow of tears nor of semen is essential to life or health. Both are largely under the control of the imagination, the emotions, and the will; and the flow of either is liable to be arrested in a moment of sudden mental action."

Parkhurst says: "The prostatic fluid, according to Robin, is secreted at the moment of ejaculation. The remaining element of the spermatic secretion is produced, under normal circumstances, only as required, either for impregnation or for the maintenance of the affectional function. The theory that the sperm is naturally secreted only as it is required, brings it into harmony with other secretions. The tears, the saliva, and the perspiration, are always required in small quantities, and the secretion is continuous; but if required in great quantities, the secretion becomes great almost instantly. The mother's milk is chiefly secreted just as it is required for the infant, and when not required the secretion entirely ceases; yet it recommences the moment the birth of another child makes it necessary. * * * A man accustomed to abstinence will not suffer from any accumulation of secretions, while a man whose absorbing glands have never had occasion to take up the secretions will be in trouble; just as a dairy cow which has not been milked will be in trouble, though if running wild she would never have any necessity for milking. * * * The objection that man needs physical relief from a continuous secretion is answered by the admitted fact that men not deficient in sexual vigor live for months, and probably for years, in strict abstinence, and with no physical inconvenience such as is often complained of by men who happen to be deprived of their accustomed indulgence for a week or two at a time."

Dr. Nystrom, the eminent Swedish writer on the subject, however, utters the following warning to those who would make hasty generalizations on the subject: "In speaking of relative abstinence or regulation and command of the sexual instinct, I warn against absolutism in this regard, and especially against the generalizing of abstinence as possible for everybody. Although abstinence during an entire lifetime does not injure certain individuals, it cannot be endured by others for some length of time without undesirable consequences. I therefore oppose the principle of absolute continence as in the main false. It may possibly be applied to a few deeply religious or philosophical persons, but not to the majority of normal people, despite good resolutions and habits. * * * We must consider the different bodily constitutions and passions—why some people without difficulty, others with the greatest difficulty, can master their feelings regarding sexual relations. * * * May those who try to better humanity in sexual respects first give their attention to the subject when well prepared with a rich experience and deep study, for otherwise they cannot give advice which can be followed, and their work should fail as being contrary to human nature."

Temporary Continence. Many married couples who are desirous of preventing too-frequent conception, or conception following too soon after the birth of the youngest child, practice the method of refraining from the marital sexual relations during certain periods in which conception is most likely to occur. This custom is said to be favored by those acting under the advice of their religious instructors, and who regard all methods of birth-control other than continence as sinful. Even the most orthodox objectors to birth-control as a general principle seem to regard this particular method as free from objection, providing that the married couple do not seek to entirely escape parenthood in this manner.

This plan is based upon the well-known, and well-established physiological principle that **the time immediately before the menstrual period, and still more, immediately after the period is the most favorable to conception**. Impregnation is most likely to occur just after the menstrual period; while from about two weeks after the beginning of the period, to a few days before the beginning of the next period, is the time of comparative sterility when impregnation and conception are the least likely to occur. Consequently, the authorities hold that the period of from ten to fifteen days after the **end** of the menstruation is one peculiarly free from the probability of impregnation and conception.

This plan of temporary continence, continuing during the period in which conception is most probable, and terminating when that period has passed each month, until the new period approaches, is followed by many married couples with the full approval of the conscience and their religious guides. In many cases the result fulfills the expectations, though as there is a considerable variation observed among different women there is no absolute certainty to the plan considered as a birth-control method—at the best it is but taking advantage of the law of probabilities, the chances being in favor of the result sought.

Semi-Continence.

Semi-Continence (in the sense in which the term is employed herein) consists of the abstinence from the exercise of the procreative functions, while there is a partial manifestation of the sexual relation. Under various fanciful names, backed by as many curious theories, this birth-control method is practiced by very many married couples in this and other countries.

Among the earlier advocates of this general class of birth-control methods was Noyes, the founder of the one-time famous Oneida Community, who taught the doctrine of what he called "Male Continence." The gist of his teaching was as follows: That the sexual relation (in its entirety) should be exercised solely for the purpose of reproduction, all else being contrary to nature. But, he held, notwithstanding this, there was possible and proper a certain degree of such physical relation which, while not opposing Nature's laws of reproduction, yet was sufficient to afford a complete manifestation of the "affectional desire and function." In other words, as a writer has expressed it, "that one might manifest a marked degree of sexual gratification and still remain continent, while feeling none of the irksome restraints of continence."

Noyes claimed that his community followed this plan with satisfactory results, the ordinary sexual relations being manifested only when reproduction was specially desired and deliberately decided upon. Noyes claimed that in this way there was no secretion of the seminal fluid, and therefore no waste of the same, and no unnatural practices such attached to the common custom of "tricking Nature" by methods of preventing impregnation and conception. Parkhurst (who, as we shall see presently, followed Noyes) objected to the Noyes plan, claiming that "it necessarily stimulates into activity the generative functions of the sexual batteries, and this not only causes a wasteful use of sperm, but diverts the sexual batteries from their affectional function, diminishing amative attraction."

In the year 1896, Dr. Alice B. Stockham, of Chicago, published a book called "Karezza" which has since attained an enormous sale, the leading principle of which seems to have been almost similar to that of Noyes, as above stated. The book was built around the idea previously announced by the same author in an earlier book, which she stated as follows: "By some a theory called 'secular absorption' is advanced. This involves intercourse without culmination." In her book "Karezza" this author further stated: "Karezza so consummates marriage that through the power of will, and loving thoughts, the crisis is not reached, but a complete control by both husband and wife is maintained throughout the entire relation, a conscious conservation of the creative energy. * * * It is both a union on the affectional plane, and a preparation for the best possible conditions for procreation."

About 1882, Henry M. Parkhurst published a booklet called "Diana," which since that time has passed through several editions, and has had a large number of readers. The principle advocated is radically different from that of Noyes or Dr. Stockham, above mentioned, although some of the writings of Dr. Stockham seem to favor the Parkhurst idea as much as the one advanced by herself. Parkhurst, as we may see by reference to a quotation from him in connection with the Noyes' idea, did not approve of the "male continence" as taught by the latter, although he seems to have considered it a step in the right direction.

The gist of the Parkhurst idea is expressed in the following quotations from his booklet, "Diana": "In order to secure proper and durable relations between the sexes, it is necessary to live in harmony with the law of Alphism, that is **abstinence except for procreation**. But if that principle is adopted alone, no means being taken to provide for the due exercise of the sexual faculties, it will likely be abandoned or lead to a life of asceticism. In order to make Alphism practicable for ordinary men and women, another law has to be observed, that is, the law of **sexual satisfaction from sexual contact**; understanding by the term 'contact' not merely physical external contact, but using the term in its more general sense to include sexual companionship, or even correspondence, bringing the minds into mental contact. The observance of this law will lead to complete and enduring satisfaction in abstinence.

"It is an observed fact that contact incites to activity the affectional action, * * * extending over the whole frame, and by their activities satisfies them, without calling into action the special generative function of the generative organs. And it is also an observed fact that the repression of this affectional activity naturally creates a desire for the exercise of the other; so that a true remedy for sexual intemperance is the full satisfaction of the affectional mode of activity by frequent and free sexual contact. Sexual satisfaction may be obtained by personal presence, conversation, a clasp of the hands, kissing, caressing, embracing, personal contact with or without the intervention of dress.

"The exercise of the affectional function tends to satiety and exhaustion in the same way as all other physical or mental exercise; but if it is not carried to excess it is a permanent benefit. * * * The principle of Alphism will tend to diminish prostitution, not only by diminishing sexual intemperance, even if the principle is not at once accepted in practice to the full extent, thus diminishing the temptation of the present generation, and the hereditary temptation of future generations; but also by correcting the physiological error which has led astray so many, i. e., that total abstinence is not conducive to health, or to the highest physical pleasure, but that the ordinary physical relation is an essential feature in male existence.

"To avoid misapprehension, these two theories should be clearly defined and the distinction between them explained. The doctrine of Alphism is confined to one principle, i. e., **the law of abstinence except for procreation**. Those who believe in this doctrine may be divided into different classes. Some believe in it as a matter of duty, to be enforced by precept and self-denial; and some believe in it as a matter of right, requiring no self-denial. In the latter is included the doctrine of 'Diana,' which may be defined as **the law of sexual satisfaction from sexual contact**. In other words, Dianism is Alphism as the result of sexual equilibration."

The general idea of Parkhurst, and those who have followed his teachings in some modified or adapted form, may be said to be based upon the following general proposition: That there is a dual function in the sexual relations, which may be stated as follows: (1) the function exercised from purely physiological causes, and which expresses the desire for the relation resulting in procreation; and (2) the function exercised from emotional causes, and which expresses what may be called the "affectional desire," i. e., the desire for the embrace, caress, fondling, and general companionship with the loved one of the other sex.

The first one of these phases, i. e., the reproductive function, is manifested by the lower animals as well as by man, and is elemental and primitive in character. It is often manifested by man without the accompaniment of the affectional function, and at times seems to be almost entirely divorced from the idea of high human affection. The second one of these phases, i. e., the affectional function, usually accompanied the procreative function in the human sexual relation, at least in the highest forms of that relation. But also, it may be and often is manifested independently of the procreative function by men and women of refinement. In fact, it would seem to be the form of physical attraction accompanying the very highest phase of love, particularly in women.

It is this affectional function which is manifested by betrothed lovers in their beautiful period of mutual understanding, sympathy, and affection. It is that characteristic of the courting days which is so precious to the woman, but which is too often sadly missed by the wife after the honeymoon. It exists often before the fires of passion are kindled, and it persists often after the flame of passion has died away. It is the expression of the purest love of youth, and of the tenderest affection of age. It is this form of sexual relation, physical though it may be, that is the outgrowth of evolution in man. May it not be that in this way man has "improved upon the sexual habits of the animals"; and that when man violates the natural restrictions held sacred by animal life, and indulges in excessive sexual relations in and out of season, that he is really manifesting a degenerative tendency instead of taking an upward step on the evolutionary scale.

There have been many excellent authorities who have held that this affectional function, and its manifestation, is far better calculated to satisfy the sexual instincts of advanced men and women than is the ordinary physical sexual relation. They claim that in the higher form of this affectional relation is to be found the secret of the joy, bliss, and happiness of the betrothed lovers, which alas! too often disappear when the other form of the relation is manifested, particularly when manifested to excess in the manner customary to so many married men. They claim that in the recognition of this fact of human life and love is to be found the secret of married happiness between wedded advanced and cultured individuals. They assert that the experience of the race, rightly considered and understood, full proves this contention.

Edward Carpenter has the following to say on this point: "It is a matter of common experience that the unrestrained outlet of the purely physical desire leaves the nature drained of its higher love-forces. * * * There are grounds for believing in the transmutability of the various forms of the passion, and grounds for thinking that the sacrifice of a lower phase may sometimes be the only condition on which a higher and more durable phase can be attained; and that, therefore, restraint (which is absolutely necessary at times) has its compensation. Anyone who has once realized how glorious a thing love is in its essence, and how indestructible, will hardly need to call anything that leads to it a sacrifice; and he is indeed a master of life who, accepting the grosser desires as they come to his body, and not refusing them, knows how to transform them at will into the most rare and fragrant flowers of human emotion * * * Between lovers, then, a kind of hardy temperance is to be recommended—for all reasons, but especially because it lifts their satisfaction and delight in each other out of the regions of ephemeralities (which too often turn into dull indifference and satiety) into the region of more lasting things—one step nearer at any rate to the eternal kingdom.

"How intoxicating, indeed, how penetrating—like a most precious wine—is that love which is the sexual transformed by the magic of the will into the emotional and spiritual! And what a loss, on the merest ground of prudence and the economy of pleasure, is the unbridled waste along physical channels! So nothing is so much dreaded between lovers as just this—the vulgarization of love—and this is the rock upon which marriage so often splits. There is a kind of illusion about physical desire similar to that which a child suffers from when, seeing a beautiful flower, it instantly snatches the same and destroys in a few moments the form and fragrance which attracted it. He only gets the full glory who holds back a little, and he only truly possesses who is willing if need be not to possess. * * * It must be remembered, however, that in order for a perfect intimacy between two people their physical endearment must by the nature of the case be free to each other. The physical endearment may not be the object for which they come together; but, if it is denied, its denial will bar any real sense of repose and affiance, and make their mutual association restless, vague, tentative and unsatisfied. I think, from various considerations, that, generally, even without the actual physical sex-act, there is an interchange of vital and ethereal elements—so that it may be said that there is a kind of generation taking place within each of the persons concerned, through their mutual influence on each other, as well as that more specialized generation which consists in the propagation of the race."

Count Tolstoi said on this subject: "The difference in organization between man and woman is not only physiological but extends also into other and moral characteristics, such as go to make manhood in man, and womanhood (or femininity) in woman. The attraction between the sexes is based not merely upon the yearning for physical union, but likewise upon that reciprocal attraction exerted by the contrasting qualities of the sexes each upon the other, manhood upon womanhood, and womanhood upon manhood. The one sex endeavors to complement itself with the other, and therefore the attraction between the sexes demands a union of spirit precisely identical with the physical union.

"The tendency toward physical and spiritual union forms two phases of manifestation of one and the same fountain-head of desire, and they bear such intimate relations to each other that the gratification of the one inclination inevitably weakens the other. So far as the yearning for spiritual union is satisfied, to that extent the yearning for physical union is diminished or entirely destroyed; and, vice versa, the gratification of the physical desire weakens or destroys the spiritual. And, consequently, the attraction between the sexes is not only physical affinity leading to procreation, but is also the attraction of opposites for one another, capable of assuming the form of the most spiritual union in thought only, or of the most animal union, causing the propagation of children, and all those varied degrees of relationship between the one and the other. The question of upon which footing the relation between the sexes is to be established and maintained, is settled by deciding what method of union is regarded at any given time, or for all time, as good, proper, and therefore desirable. * * *

"The nearer the union approaches the extreme physical boundary, the more it kindles the physical passions and desires, and the less satisfaction it gets; the nearer it approaches the opposite extreme spiritual boundary, the less new passions are excited and the greater is the satisfaction. The nearer it is to the first, the more destructive it is to animal energy; the nearer it approaches the second, the spiritual, the more serene, the more enjoyable and forceful is the general condition. * * * Taking into consideration the varying conditions of temperament, and above all what the contracting parties regard as good, proper, and desirable, marriage for some will approach the spiritual union, and for others the physical; but the nearer the union approaches the spiritual the more complete will be the satisfaction. The substance of what has been said is this: that the relation between the sexes have two functions, i. e., the reproductive, and the affectional; and that the sexual energy, if only it have no conscious desire to beget children, must be always directed in the way of affection and love. The manifestation which this energy assumes depends upon custom or reason; the gradual bringing of the reason into accord with the principles herein expounded, and a gradual reorganization of customs consonant with them, results in saving men from many of their passions, and giving them satisfaction for their higher sexual instincts and desires."

Some capable writers on the subject have held that in the practice of the methods of semi-continence, such as have been referred to in the foregoing pages of this part of the book, there may lie the danger of excessive stimulation of the sexual centres, without the safety-valve of the physical and nervous relief which follows as a natural sequence in the ordinary sexual relations. The advocates of these methods, however, reply that such objections while valid in the case of persons who practice the same only because opportunity prevents the performance of the usual physical relation, still have no true application to those who adopt these methods in a conscientious and honest manner, and who maintain **the proper mental attitude** toward the whole question.

These advocates say that the **mental effect** upon the secretions of the body must be taken into account in all considerations of the question. They say that just as the gastric juice will begin to flow in response to the mental image or idea of food, and the mother's milk in response to the cry of the child for food, so do the sexual secretions, direction of the circulation, and other physiological activities result from the mental pictures or idea of sexual congress. They hold that if the mind of the husband be filled with mental images of sexual congress, then there is set into operation the process of secretion of seminal fluids, and the consequent engorgement of the blood-vessels concerned therewith, which are denied the normal physiological relief, and accordingly produce bad effects upon the nervous system. But they likewise claim that if the mind of the husband entertains ideas merely of physical endearment and caress as "an end to itself," then there is no mental incentive toward the secretion of the seminal fluids, and the constant engorgement of the blood-vessels, and no nerve force is generated—and therefore no nerve-shock is experienced by reason of frustrated manifestation and expression.

Parkhurst says regarding the point just mentioned: "In the relations between the sexes, the question of how the association of the husband and the wife shall stimulate the affectional or generative action or sexual batteries must depend greatly upon their habits of association. We have only to accustom ourselves to associating the relation with the affectional action, by repeated repetition when the affectional action is all that is felt or thought of, in order to cultivate such habits and associations as will make the association tend to **repress** passional desires, by the direction of the sexual forces into the channel of affectional attraction and functioning. * * * The form of the sexual manifestation will be largely influenced, by the mind, and largely by force with these principles, and the gradual formation of habits consistent therewith, will make more and more evident their beneficial operation."

There is much interest now being taken by thinking people in some phases of the general subject of semi-continence, and many thoughtful and conscientious persons find in it at least the promise of a worthy and honest solution of the problem of Continence as applied to Birth Control. Such persons claim to find in this general class of Birth Control methods a happy medium between the rigid practice of absolute Continence in the marriage relations, on the one hand, and the more popular methods of Contraception, on the other hand.

Contraception.

We now come to the consideration of the subject of Contraception, pure and simple, the methods of which contemplate the manifestation of the usual physical sexual relations between husband and wife, accompanied by an avoidance of the union of the male and female elements of reproduction which result in conception.

It should once more be positively emphasized that **by Contraception is NOT meant Abortion. Abortion** means "the premature expulsion of the human embryo or foetus; miscarriage." **Contraception**, on the other hand, means simply the prevention of the union of the male and female elements of reproduction, and consequently, the preventing of the process which evolves the foetus or embryo. **Contraception is prevention; abortion is destruction.** There is here a difference as wide as the poles. As Dr. William J. Robinson says, in a paragraph previously quoted in this book: "In inducing abortion, one destroys something already formed—a foetus, or an embryo, a fertilized ovum, a potential human being. In prevention, however, one merely prevents chemically or mechanically the spermatozoa from coming in contact with the ovum. There is no greater sin or crime in this than there is in simple abstinence, in refraining from sexual intercourse."

Unfortunately for the cause of scientific Birth Control in America, the laws of the United States (and of most of the separate States) at present prevent the public dissemination by written or printed words, or by public teaching of information concerning the contraceptive methods known to all intelligent physicians and others who have made a scientific study of the subject. The conveyal of such information, in the manner stated, is made a criminal offence, subject to heavy fines and imprisonment. Though there is a strong movement underway on the part of many intelligent and earnest citizens of this country, having for its object the repeal of such prohibitive laws, and the passage of careful legislation designed to give the dissemination of such instruction a legal and certain status, under the restrictions imposed by common sense, intellectual honesty, and the best interests of the race—to place it upon the same footing as in certain advanced European countries—the fact remains that at the present time no person may give such information without subjecting himself to indictment and probable conviction as a law-breaker and enemy of society. **Under the circumstances, of course, there has been, and will be, no attempts to furnish such forbidden information in this book.** So long as these laws stand unrepealed on the statute books, they must be observed by all law abiding citizens.

Dr. Wm. J. Robinson, an authority on the subject, says: "We believe that under any conditions, and particularly under our present economic conditions, human beings should be able to control the number of their offspring. They should be able to decide how many children they want to have, and when they want to have them. And to accomplish this result we demand that the knowledge of controlling the number of offspring, in other and plainer words, the knowledge of preventing undesirable conception, should not be considered a criminal offence punishable by hard labor in Federal prisons, but that it should be considered knowledge useful and necessary to the welfare of the race and of the individual; and that its dissemination should be as permissible as is the dissemination of any hygienic, sanitary or eugenic knowledge."

The only possible relief from the present condition is seen by careful thinkers to be in the education of the public as to the needs of the case, and the presentation of the scientific argument in favor of rational and proper Birth Control, to the end that public opinion, once seeing the truth in the case, may be sufficiently strong as to bring about a change in the present antiquated and bigoted laws. But, so long as the laws remain on the statute books, they must be observed and obeyed. Education, not Anarchy, is the true remedy.

The following general remarks on the subject of Contraception, by Havelock Ellis, the well-known English authority of the subject of Sex in Modern Society, may perhaps prove interesting to students of the general subject: Ellis says: "Many ways of preventing conception have been devised since the method which is still the commonest was first introduced, so far as our certainly imperfect knowledge extends, by a clever Jew, Onan (Genesis, Chap. XXXVIII) whose name has since been wrongly attached to another practice with which the Mosaic record in no way associates him. There are now many contraceptive methods, some dependent on precautions adopted by the man, others dependent upon the woman, others again which take the form of an operation permanently preventing conception, and, therefore, not to be adopted save by couples who already have as many children as they desire, or else who ought never to have children at all and thus wisely adopt a method of sterilization. It is unnecessary here, even if it were otherwise desirable, to discuss these various methods in detail. It is even useless to do so, for we must bear in mind that no method can be absolutely approved or absolutely condemned. Each may be suitable under certain conditions and for certain couples, and it is not easy to recommend any method indiscriminately. We need to know the intimate circumstances of individual cases. For the most part, experience is the final test.

"Forel compared the use of contraceptive devices to the use of eyeglasses, and it is obvious that, without expert advice, the results in either case may sometimes be mischievous or at all events ineffective. Personal advice and instruction are always desirable. In Holland nurses are medically trained in a practical knowledge of contraceptive methods, and are thus enabled to enlighten the women of the community. This is an admirable plan. Considering that the use of contraceptive measures is now almost universal, it is astonishing that there are yet so many 'civilized' countries in which this method of enlightenment is not everywhere adopted. Until it is adopted, and a necessary knowledge of the most fundamental facts of sexual life brought into every home, the physician must be regarded as the proper adviser. It is true that until recently he was generally in these matters a blind leader of the blind. Nowadays it is beginning to be recognized that the physician has no more serious and responsible duty than that of giving help in the difficult path of sexual life. Very frequently, indeed, even yet, he has not risen to a sense of his responsibilities in this matter. It is well to remember, however, that a physician who is unable or unwilling to give frank and sound advice in this most important department of life, is unlikely to be reliable in any other department. If he is not up to date here, he is probably not up to date anywhere.

"Whatever may be the method adopted, there are certain conditions which it must fulfill, even apart from its effectiveness as a contraceptive, in order to be satisfactory. Most of these conditions may be summed up in one: the most satisfactory method is that which least interferes with the normal process in the act of intercourse. Every sexual act is, or should be, a miniature courtship, however long marriage may have lasted. No outside mental tension or nervous apprehension must be allowed to intrude. Any contraceptive proceeding which hastily enters the atmosphere of love immediately before or immediately after the moment of union is unsatisfactory and may be injurious. It even risks the total loss of the contraceptive result, for at such moments the intended method may be ineffectively carried out, or neglected altogether. No method can be regarded as desirable which interferes with the sense of satisfaction and relief which should follow the supreme act of loving union. No method which produces a nervous jar in one of the parties, even though it may be satisfactory to the other, should be tolerated. Such considerations must for some couples rule out certain methods. We cannot, however, lay down absolute rules, because methods some couples may find satisfactory prove unsatisfactory in other cases. Experience, aided by expert advice, is the only final criterion.

"When a contraceptive method is adopted under satisfactory conditions, with a due regard to the requirements of the individual couple, there is little room to fear that any injurious results will be occasioned. It is quite true that many physicians speak emphatically concerning the injurious results to husband or to wife of contraceptive devices. Although there has been exaggeration, and prejudice has often been imported into this question, and although most of the injurious results could have been avoided had trained medical help been at hand to advise better methods, there can be no doubt that much that has been said under this head is true. Considering how widespread is the use of these methods, and how ignorantly they have often been carried out, it would be surprising indeed if it were not true. But even supposing that the nervously injurious effects which have been traced to contraceptive practices were a thousandfold greater than they have been reported to be—instead of, as we are justified in believing, considerably less than they are reported—shall we therefore condemn contraceptive methods? To do so would be to ignore all the vastly greater evils which have followed in the past from unchecked reproduction. It would be a condemnation which, if we exercised it consistently, would destroy the whole of civilization and place us back in savagery. For what device of man, ever since man had any history at all, has not proved sometimes injurious?

"Every one of even the most useful and beneficial of human inventions has either exercised subtle injuries or produced appalling catastrophes. This is not only true of man's devices, it is true of Nature's in general. Let us take, for instance, the elevation of man's ancestors from the quadrupedal to the bipedal position. The experiment of making a series of four-footed animals walk on their hind-legs was very evolutionary and risky; it was far more beset by dangers than is the introduction of contraceptives; we are still suffering all sorts of serious evils in consequence of Nature's action in placing our remote ancestors in the erect position. Yet we feel that it was worth while; even those physicians who most emphasize the evil results of the erect position do not advise that we should go on all-fours. It is just the same with a great human device, the introduction of clothes. They have led to all sorts of new susceptibilities to disease and even tendencies to direct injury of many kinds. Yet no one advocates the complete disuse of all clothing on the ground that corsets have sometimes proved harmful. It would be just as absurd to advocate the complete abandonment of contraceptives on the ground that some of them have been misused. If it were not, indeed, that we are familiar with the lengths to which ignorance and prejudice may go we should question the sanity of anyone who put forward so foolish a proposition. Every great step which Nature and man have taken in the path of progress has been beset by dangers which are gladly risked because of the advantages involved. We must never loose sight of the immense advantages which Man has gained in acquiring a conscious and deliberate control of reproduction."

THE END.

Milton Keynes UK
Ingram Content Group UK Ltd.
UKHW051056220424
441551UK00015B/1046

9 781805 478133